FORMULA *for* LIFE

Formula for Life

Revised Edition

Eberhard Kronhausen, Ed.D.,

and

Phyllis Kronhausen, Ed.D.

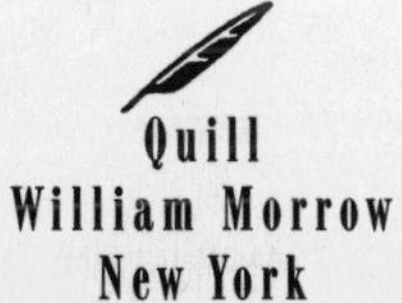

Quill
William Morrow
New York

Before beginning this or any other nutritional regimen, consult a nutrition-oriented physician to be sure it is medically appropriate for you.

The information in this book is not intended to replace medical advice. Any medical questions, general or specific, should be addressed to your physician.

It is the policy of William Morrow and Company, Inc., and its imprints and affiliates, recognizing the importance of preserving what has been written, to print the books we publish on acid-free paper, and we exert our best efforts to that end.

Library of Congress Cataloging-in-Publication Data

Kronhausen, Eberhard, 1915–
Formula for Life / Eberhard Kronhausen and Phyllis Kronhausen.—rev. ed.
p. cm.
Includes bibliographical references and index.
ISBN 0-688-15123-X (alk. paper)
1. Dietary supplements. 2. Nutrition. 3. Vitamins.
4. Antioxidants—health aspects. 5. Longevity—nutritional aspects. I. Kronhausen, Phyllis, 1929– . II. Title.
RA784.K76 1999
613.2—dc21 98–49386
CIP

Printed in the United States of America

First Edition

1 2 3 4 5 6 7 8 9 10

BOOK DESIGN BY MERYL SUSSMAN LEVAVI/DIGITEXT, INC.

www.williammorrow.com

Foreword

As a practicing physician with a *very* traditional background, I have spent many years watching the successes and failures of traditional medical treatment. We in the West have made enormous strides over the last one hundred years in the treatment of some types of illnesses, including infectious diseases and trauma—the kinds of problems that arise quickly can kill you in short order and, if treated properly, can result in almost miraculous recoveries. Unfortunately, though, our success with these types of illnesses has blinded us, to some degree, and led us in the "traditional," "scientific," or "allopathic" schools of medicine to believe that we may be able to treat all diseases, illnesses, and disorders of the body and mind similarly, with a single "magic bullet," analogous to antibiotics. "If only we can find the single crucial biochemical causation of this disease," we reason, "we can devise a treatment or cure." Such reasoning is sometimes correct and proper, but many times chronic disorders have many, many causative factors, and therefore lend themselves to many, many different approaches for prevention and treatment. More information concerning our successes has led, in many instances, to a severe case of "N.I.H. syndrome" (Not Invented Here).

In the case of medical treatment, this goes something like: "If Western, allopathic, traditional medicine doesn't know about disease, or treatment, or preventative measures, then it probably doesn't exist, is just 'quackery,' or at the very least certainly doesn't deserve serious attention. After all, if it were important, we would be looking into it. . . ."

This type of circular reasoning kept antisepsis from being

accepted for decades, led to most amputations during the Civil War being performed without anesthesia (even though it had been demonstrated successfully at the Massachusetts General Hospital nearly twenty years earlier), and ridiculed an obscure Australian physician who discovered the cause of most cases of gastric ulceration twenty-five years ago, until the evidence became so overwhelming that even the "experts" accepted it.

The scientific approach is the right one, but we practitioners and physicians *must* keep an open mind, *must* look at all evidence for illnesses and their treatment impartially, and *must* be willing to change our assumptions when the findings don't fit them. Clearly, we in the medical profession don't have a monopoly on knowledge or scientific expertise, and we should remember that.

Drs. Eberhard and Phyllis Kronhausen have compiled, in this fascinating volume, very important confirmations of the benefit of many types of "nontraditional" approaches to health maintenance. As in their first volume, careful documentation of research is the rule, and presentation of firsthand accounts of interactions with active patients and practitioners makes for interesting reading. Perhaps most refreshing for me, a practitioner, is the fact that much of the information comes from sources which feel comfortable and familiar. Journal articles, interviews with practicing physicians, and firsthand information—all are important sources for making up one's mind about the efficacy, or benefit, of a particular approach to a disorder. As important as the information, though, in my opinion, is the clear and open presentation, and the tolerant approach. The authors state it best: "You will be informed and able to make up your own mind."

The Kronhausens remind us, both directly and subtly, to always, *always* remember several things. The health care practitioner you see is not your father or mother (in all probability), is certainly not God, and has his or her own beliefs, justifications, and prejudices. The *only* person you can trust with your health, just like the *only* person you can trust with anything else you value, is *you*. You must become informed. You must question your doctors, your ancillary health-care practitioners, and your information sources. You must seek to understand whatever problem besets you and make your own decisions concerning what to do about it. The information presented in the revised edition of *Formula for Life* may be an excellent introduction to many new and interesting ideas for those who are lost in the almost impenetrable thicket of medical information. Sometimes presenting many of these ideas to a nonmedical audience can be difficult, especially when they may not be "mainstream," but the Kronhausens manage it admirably. Their chapters on Dr. Nagourney, and on the importance of "attitudinal adjustment" as an adjunct to successful treatment of serious illness, will give both hope and information to many afflicted with disorders that may be life-threatening.

To all my fellow practitioners, I urge—read it! Even if the ideas seem foreign, or do not fit into your traditional style of thinking, use it as a reference resource for information concerning some of the most important topics your patients will want to discuss with you! To patients and interested family members, I urge the same—read the book, and take it with you to your physician. Ask questions, demand explanations, and make sure you understand before you make a decision. Knowledge is power.

—Timothy Kaiser, M.D., F.A.C.S.

Foreword

It is now recognized that 60 percent of women's cancers and 40 percent of men's cancers are nutritionally related. Drs. Eberhard and Phyllis Kronhausen have thoroughly reviewed the benefits of nutritional factors that will aid in preventing diseases and help those who do have illnesses.

Cancer will emerge as the number one cause of death in the United States by the year 2000. Despite the enormous effort to combat cancer, the number of new cases of nearly every form of cancer has increased annually over the last century. Still worse: From 1930 to the present, despite the introduction of radiation therapy, chemotherapy, and immunotherarpy with biological response modifiers, CT scans, MR scans, and all other new medical technology, lifespans for almost every form of adult cancer except cervical cancer and lung cancer have remained constant, which means that there has been no significant progress in cancer treatment. The successes in the treatment of cancer plateaued in the 1970s, and no real advances have been made since then. However, chemotherapy and radiation therapy continue to have a role in cancer treatment—yet they produce morbidity. Nutritional modification, including the use of certain nutrients, and a proper lifestyle can dramatically decrease the morbidity and side effects of chemotherapy and radiation therapy while at the same time increasing the response rates of those modalities. There have been some reports that nutritional and lifestyle modification actually increase survival.

The Drs. Kronhausen have done a great service for you in organizing nutritional information and mind-body relationships. This revised edition of *Formula for Life* should be part of everyone's library as a resource against disease.

—Charles B. Simone, M.D., author of *Cancer and Nutrition, Breast Health*, and *Shark Cartilage and Cancer*

Acknowledgments

If this book reads as well as we think it does, the credit and thanks go primarily to our friend and private editor, Hubert B. Herring, a writer and editor with *The New York Times*. Much of an earlier version was lovingly edited by our friend Diana Palm. These two wondeful and patient people, Hubert and Diana, made sure that none of Eberhard's occasional lapses into German sentence structure sneaked into the manuscript.

Aside from that, we wish to express our deeply felt gratitude to two very special friends whose generosity kept us alive through the last year of working on this book: Rodrigo Arias, former Minister of the Presidency and current President of the Stock Exchange in Costa Rica, and our good neighbor Dr. Fred Greiner, also of Costa Rica. Without their financial help, we would not have been able to dedicate ourselves almost full-time to the research and writing of this book.

Special thanks also to Chet and Linda Augustine, who let us share their spacious SoHo loft with them and put up with the mess of our many books and ever-growing piles of research papers, which often left hardly an empty place on their dining table.

There is one other friend to whom we want to express our special thanks: Michael Wright, software specialist and programmer at New York University's Multi-Media department and our faithful "computer guru." He always came to our rescue, as nobody else would have done, whenever our "functional illiteracy" about computers got us into a tight spot and threatened to paralyze our work.

Last but not least, we want to thank Robert A. Nagourney,

M.D., for generously giving us of his scarce time and allowing us to interview him at such great length about his unique approach to the treatment of cancer. The same goes for our interview with Giovanna Casola, M.D., at the time, one of the country's foremost experts on the bloodless technique of Cryosurgery for prostate cancer. And equal thanks to our good friend, Milos Sovak, M.D., President of Biophysica, a private biomedical research institute in La Jolla, California, for introducing us to Dr. Casola and for befriending us in many other ways.

Likewise, we are grateful to microbiologist Alan H. Kapuler, Ph.D., for permission to include his illuminating personal experiences with the healing potential of macrobiotics, even in the case of serious cancer.

In either case, the only goal of these scientists clearly was to selflessly share their vast and maybe life-saving knowledge and experiences with you, the reader, and for the benefit of the general public.

Contents

PART SIX
"FRIENDLY" FOODS 149

PART SEVEN
"UNFRIENDLY" FOODS 219

Letter to the Reader

Dear friend:

Forgive us for taking the liberty of addressing you as "friend" even though we haven't met—not in the normal way, at any rate. Yet you obviously share our interest in health, and in slowing down the life-span clock. If you didn't, you wouldn't have picked up this book, right? So we have a lot in common, and common interests are the strongest bonds. It is in this sense that we think of you as a friend—and hope that you will do likewise.

Perhaps you already know us from the original edition of *Formula for Life* (William Morrow, 1989). If so, consider that volume a good introduction to the one you now hold in your hands. If not, don't be concerned; this book requires no introductory reading.

Many things we talk about here, though, are based on the same scientific principles we discussed more fully in our earlier book—like the free radical theory of disease and ageing, and the role that antioxidants can play in counteracting the destructive, life-shortening effects of these abnormal molecules.

In that sense, this book picks up where our earlier one left off. So we will not tell you again what the common vitamins—like B, C, and E—are good for. Chances are you take them already. But in addition to reiterating that only the right combinations and dosages make them really therapeutic, we want to explain their less well understood immunity-enhancing and life-extending properties.

Nor do we intend to bore you with admonitions about diet that you can read anywhere, except to give you a few warnings about some "unfriendly" foods that you might never suspect. But we will also introduce you to some wonderful, "friendly" foods you may not know about.

In addition, we want to tell you about some powerful new antioxidants discovered in recent years—like coenzyme Q-10 and L-carnitine, both of which turn out to be very important to keep our hearts ticking; and alpha lipoic acid, which has tremendous antioxidant power in both the watery and fat-containing parts of our cells and helps prevent or control diabetes.

You should also know about the important pycnogenols (technically, proanthocyanidins); natural substances in pine bark and grape seeds. They are important antioxidants frequently overlooked in this country, but used in Europe for years in the natural treatment of circulatory problems, such as varicose veins, edema, and the dangerous clumping of platelets in arteries that can cause heart attack and stroke.

We must also tell you of natural plant antioxidants like curcumin, from the spice turmeric, and lycopene, a compound in tomatoes, which protects against prostate cancer. You should also know about boswellia, the Ayurvedic, anti-inflammatory tree resin from India, which, together with glucosamine and chondroitin, is undoubtedly the best thing there is for arthritis and other inflammatory diseases—and with fewer side effects, if any, than pharmaceutical anti-inflammatory drugs.

Aside from all this, we'll discuss the controversy over hormones like melatonin, DHEA, and pregnenolone. As you may know, some doctors are dead-set against people taking these hormones, while others, like the renowned oncologist and endocrinologist Dr. William Regelson (author of *The Superhormone Promise*), are all for having older folks like us, whose hormone levels are usually in the subbasement, take hormone supplements.

Chances are you don't know whether to believe the "yea-sayers" or "nay-sayers" on this subject; we have been confused about it, too. So we've gone right to the scientific sources and spent hundreds of hours in medical libraries to see for ourselves which of the two camps had more science on its side.

We shall give you a summary of what we learned about these hormones, why we decided, in the end, to use them, and what our own experience with them has been. That way you'll be fully informed and able to make up your own mind on this important issue. On the other hand, we certainly don't approve of people blithely taking these supplements without monitoring of hormone levels. (The only trouble is that many doctors have not followed the latest research, so you have to be careful about whom to consult.)

We also want to introduce you to two brilliant and truly "different" cancer specialists at the very cutting edge of medical science and practice, because knowing about them might, some day, be vital to you or to someone you care deeply about. For, let's face it, one in three or four of us will come face to face with the "Big C," to use Susan Sontag's shorthand term.

We met one of these extraordinary doctors, Robert Nagourney, M.D., some years ago in California, when Eberhard had his own close encounter with what seemed to be colon cancer. (As it turned out, Eberhard's colon tumor had not yet reached the stage of full-blown cancer. His much more serious encounter came some time later, when a malignant melanoma lesion was discovered on his hip. But, luckily again, it apparently had not yet gone too deep to be excised and, thus far, our antioxidants seem to keep it in check.)

Dr. Robert Nagourney, who became Eberhard's own doctor, does not believe in treating cancer with highly toxic chemotherapy before knowing that these drugs will really work for a particular patient. He therefore developed a highly sophisticated laboratory procedure, in which the patient's cancer cells are exposed to a variety of the usual chemotherapy drugs, as well as some unusual ones, to see whether they'll respond to any of them. If not—and, apparently, quite a few patients' cancer cells don't respond to standard chemotherapy—the doctor had better look for alternatives, says Dr. Nagourney, or the patient will be needlessly exposed to highly toxic drugs that cannot possibly do any good.

The other unusual physician we think you should know about, Giovanna Casola, M.D., specializes in prostate cancer cryosurgery, a much more benign, bloodless freezing technique than radical surgery. She successfully treated a close friend of ours, himself a medical researcher, with this advanced technique, which has a much lower incidence of incontinence and impotence, not to mention a much shorter and less painful recovery time. Yet cryosurgery and Dr. Nagourney's sensitivity test for cancer drugs rank among the medical establishment's best-kept secrets.

There is still another person we think we should introduce you to: Dr. Alan Kapuler, a microbiologist. He had consulted Dr. Nagourney because he had just been diagnosed with lymphoma, a cancer of the blood and lymphatic systems. As it turned out, Dr. Nagourney's lab test showed that about the only chemo drug that was effective against his cancer cells was also one of the most toxic ones. Dr. Kapuler, knowing what he did, as a scientist, about the devastating side effects of that particular drug, decided against chemotherapy. Instead, he opted to take his chances with something that is not even a recognized alternative cancer therapy: macrobiotics.

We will let him tell you, in his own words, how he went about using only organically grown foods, taking some herbal remedies and—last but not least, following a tranquil, relatively low-stress lifestyle in the Oregon countryside—to keep his serious case of lymphoma in long-term remission. We do not mean to say that we advocate macrobiotics as standard cancer therapy, but every once in a while somebody like Dr. Kapuler comes along and forces us to think again.

Lastly, but with no less urgency, we want to talk to you about making not only our bodies but our minds work to keep us in good health. For what is the use of taking the most powerful antioxidants, watching our diet, and working out at the gym, if the mind is undermining our health with negative thoughts and emotions?

Put differently, the way we think and relate to others and the world around us does, for better or worse, affect our physical well-being in a thousand subtle ways. When we're depressed or anxious, our immune system is down, too, and we're more sickness-prone than during happier times. We all know that; but "keeping our cool" is not so easy when the going gets rough. We'd therefore like to let you hear what some wonderfully courageous and creative people have said and done when faced with very adverse circumstances, even impending death. They have been a great inspiration to us, and we know they will be to you, as well.

So that is what this book is all about. We can only hope, dear friend, that the information it contains and the people you'll meet on these pages will be as meaningful and helpful to you as they have been to us. If you're well, may the book help you remain well; if you are ill, may it show you new and unexpected possibilities of healing both body and mind.

Cordially yours,

Eberhard Kronhausen
Phyllis Kronhausen

Part One

Laying the Foundation

Chapter 1

THE CONTROVERSY ABOUT SUPPLEMENTS

There is a continuing running battle among health professionals with regard to nutritional supplements: there are those, like us, who believe in them, and others who think they are just a "rip-off" and are doing more harm than good. Take, for instance, Jane Brody, the highly respected health columnist of *The New York Times*. She usually reports very knowledgeably and evenhandedly about matters of health and nutrition, but loses her objectivity and seems to be absolutely phobic when it comes to nutritional supplements.

There was, for example, Ms. Brody's sensationalist, and alarmist, column about the alleged dangers of vitamins and other nutritional supplements.* Starting on the paper's front page and running for a full page inside, it is one shrill warning after an-

**The New York Times,* 26 October 1997.

other about the alleged dangers of one or another vitamin, mineral, antioxidant, or amino acid—unless, of course, it is part of *food.*

In that article, as in many others, Ms. Brody presented her "personal" views about what she thinks are the risks involved in taking such supplements, at least in any but the most minimal dosages. Only that to her, everything beyond the minidoses of a few supplements, such as 400 mg of vitamin C and 200 IU (International Units) of vitamin E, along with perhaps a few hundred micrograms of folic acid that she herself takes, looks like "megadoses."

Now, that's a perfectly legitimate, personal point of view and, while it's not strictly based on science, we do respect it. But the trouble is that Ms. Brody and others like her sometimes present such opinions as if they were reporting on brand-new, objective research. In actual fact, though, all the oft-touted "dangers" from overdosing on certain specific supplements—like vitamin B-6 and vitamin A, as well as minerals like selenium and iron—have been known for years, and put in proper proportion against their health *benefits* by many writers, including ourselves.

There is also the perennial argument, proposed by supplement foes like Ms. Brody, that the vitamin-taking public are unwitting "guinea pigs" in a large-scale but uncontrolled safety study. Quite right; but that just proves the point that vitamins and similar nutritional supplements are perfectly safe when taken in sensible doses and not being abused.

We ourselves qualify as "guinea pigs," for we have, over more than fifteen years, taken what Ms. Brody would call "megadoses" (we and many other health professionals would call them *therapeutic* doses) of vitamins, minerals, and other supplements. The result? Every doctor who ever examined us says that our biological ages seems at least ten years less than our chronological ages. None of them has found any damage; quite the contrary. Some of them—all mainstream medical specialists—even credited our vitamin/antioxidant program for our remarkably good health.

But, yes—it is possible to overdose on certain vitamins and minerals, if they are grossly abused (just as some people abuse perfectly good foods and get sick from overeating).

Vitamin B-6, mentioned by Ms. Brody, is a case in point. We already discussed the potential toxicity of this vitamin, if taken in unreasonable amounts, in the earlier edition of *Formula for Life,* published in 1989—and it wasn't news, even then.

We pointed out that in the handful of such cases known to have occurred, people had taken doses far in excess of the dose in our basic vitamin/antioxidant program. Even so, no permanent harm was done; the neurological symptoms (prickling, antlike, sometimes painful sensations in hands and feet) that large overdoses of vitamin B-6 can cause, disappeared in every one of these cases, as soon as the abuse was discontinued.

Ms. Brody also calls attention to the fact that iron supplements can do more harm than good. That's absolutely true. We have always maintained that iron supplements ought not to be taken, unless in the presence of diagnosed iron deficiency, and we are repeating this warning again here. Iron overload can indeed cause serious trouble, especially for the liver. We are especially concerned about iron supplements being pushed onto women and older people. So on this point we are completely in agreement with Jane Brody.

As to very large doses of vitamin E—fifty times the standard level of 400 to 800 IU a day—possibly causing excessive bleeding, that, too, is not news. We have been taking 1,200 IU of vitamin E for many years, because vitamin E is especially good for the heart and important for preventing oxidation of vitamin C. But, obviously, one shouldn't take vitamin E by the spoonful.

Ms. Brody also mentions possible gastrointestinal irritation from too much zinc ("too much" being defined as more than 12 mg for women and 10 mg for men). Very well; we take 5 mg a day, which is the generally recommended dose. But some zinc supplementation is important, especially for men, because it protects with regard to the prostate, as we shall discuss.

Ms. Brody also discusses selenium. Yes, it is possible to overdose on this trace element. But the consensus of scientific opinion now is that its potential risks have been overblown. Here, again, our readers will find an in-depth discussion of the matter in our section on selenium.

One more thing: Ms. Brody quotes Larry Norton, M.D., of the Memorial Sloan-Kettering Cancer Center in New York, as saying that large doses of vitamin C can interfere with chemotherapy for breast cancer. Maybe so; we have all due respect for Dr. Norton, a prominent breast cancer specialist. But, as of this writing—and Dr. Norton has been saying this for over a year—he has not published any data supporting his opinion. Furthermore, other equally prominent cancer specialists like Dr. Charles Simone of the Simone Protective Cancer Center in Lawrenceville, New Jersey, disagree with Dr. Norton (in Chapter 4 we discuss whether antioxidants are compatible with cancer treatments).

While we are on the topic of vitamin C: the latest assault against it comes, again, from none other than Jane Brody of *The New York Times*. This time, Ms. Brody teamed up with—of all people—the self-appointed "quack buster" Dr. Victor Herbert, professor of medicine at the Mount Sinai School of Medicine in New York.

Given this kind of collaboration, it is not surprising that the headline on Ms. Brody's latest antisupplement missile blared the warning: "Taking Too Much Vitamin C Can Be Dangerous, Study Finds."*

We have to ask ourselves, first of all, what is this dire warning about vitamin C really based on? Where is the evidence for it?

It turns out that its only foundation is a small study by two British scientists at the University of Leicester, published in the British journal *Nature,* which normally would not arouse much professional attention.

What the two chemical pathologists actually found was, on closer look, not at all what the *New York Times* headline suggests. Rather, their six-week study of thirty healthy men and women

**The New York Times,* 9 April 1998.

showed that 500 mg of supplemental vitamin C produced an antioxidant as well as a pro-oxidant effect on human DNA. There apparently was genetic damage to one part of DNA and, simultaneously, a protective effect to another part of it. In other words, there were *offsetting trends* with regard to the effect of a 500 mg vitamin C supplement.

The net result of the study remained unclear, even to the scientists themselves. Nowhere in their published study did they say, "too much vitamin C can be dangerous."

Nonetheless—especially with a helping hand from Dr. Herbert—it was not hard for Ms. Brody to make a first-class scare story out of this bland and unpretentious report. Going well outside the scope of the study, Dr. Herbert took direct aim, not so much at vitamin C *per se* as at vitamin C supplements. "Unlike vitamin C naturally present in foods, like orange juice," he pronounced, "vitamin C as a supplement is not an antioxidant." But immediately afterward, as if realizing he had overstepped himself, Dr. Herbert toned down his own rhetoric, adding that vitamin C is a "redox agent—an antioxidant in some circumstances and a pro-oxidant in others."

That is true, but is not news. There is general agreement, as Dr. Herbert says in support of his position, that when an antioxidant like vitamin C comes into contact with metal ions like iron in the body, such contact can generate free radicals. Under these circumstances, vitamin C may indeed become a pro-oxidant. But it would be obvious to anyone, except to those as deeply prejudiced against supplements as Dr. Herbert, that this applies without regard to whether the antioxidant is synthetic or from natural sources.

If, however, one compares taking a synthetic vitamin C supplement to drinking orange juice, as Dr. Herbert does, he is comparing the incomparable. Orange juice obviously is not only vitamin C. It also contains other antioxidants like beta-carotene and B-vitamins, minerals, bioflavonoids, and so on. If the vitamin C in orange juice acts, in effect, only as an antioxidant and not also as a pro-oxidant, as Dr. Herbert seems to be saying, that would not be surprising (although we have yet to see any evidence of it). But if so, our guess would be that the other antioxidants in orange juice may prevent the vitamin C from becoming oxidized and turning into a pro-oxidant—which is exactly the reason we are so much against taking single vitamins, including vitamin C, whether synthetic or natural. (Dr. Herbert, by the way, does not seem to be aware of vitamin C supplements from natural sources, such as rose hips, which would have been a more legitimate comparison.)

Furthermore—to return to the matter of DNA damage from vitamin C—one also has to keep in mind that repair enzymes constantly "patrol" our DNA strands, snipping out damaged segments and splicing in new, healthy ones. Such genetic damage is, thus, only temporary. In addition, many studies show that vitamin C also protects against oxidative DNA damage produced within the organism by oxidizing substances like iron or hydrogen peroxide.* So this whole problem is extremely complex and cannot be reduced to simplistic statements like "too much vitamin C can be dangerous."†

But why would a minor and relatively inconsequential study like that receive so much international publicity in the first place?

For an answer we must delve into the history of this vitamin C–scare story. It originated, after all, not with *The New York Times* but with the London *Times,* which first reported on the British study. But why would that paper single out this particular study to bring to the attention of the British public?

Keep in mind that the London *Times* was tipped off about the vitamin C study not by a scientific but by a political source—a press release from the British Food Ministry.

*See, for instance, Fraga, C. G., et al. Ascorbic acid protects against endogenous oxidative DNA damage in human sperm. *Proc. Natl. Acad. Sci. USA,* 88 (24):11003–11006.

†For those interested in unbiased scientific information on vitamin C, we suggest the following recent survey: *Vitamin C in Health and Disease,* L. Packer and J. Fuchs, eds. NY: Marcel Decker (especially Chapter 17, "The Mechanisms Underlying the Action of Vitamin C in Viral and Immunodeficiency Disease").

How do we know that? Because the London *Times* article talks first about a totally unrelated matter, vitamin B-6—another favorite scarecrow of antisupplement ideologues—which we discussed earlier. It said, "The government has moved to limit the use of vitamin B-6, because of safety concerns." Then, we read—and here is the clue—"Jeff Rooker, the Food Minister, had already announced that *vitamin C was his next target*" (italics ours).

It looks suspiciously as if the British Food Minister needed an excuse to "crack down" on nutritional supplements. But to do so, the Minister first had to scare the British public into believing there was a real health hazard. Without such fear-mongering, politicians and bureaucrats simply cannot get public support for their irrational interference with personal decision making.

To achieve his ends, all the British Food Minister had to do was to call the press's attention to the study in *Nature,* give it a little interpretive "spin," and—*voilà!*—out comes antivitamin propaganda that is innocently (or not-so-innocently) picked up by journalists around the world.

Take, for example, an article that appeared in California's *San Jose Mercury News*. In this case also, the journalist asked the same Dr. Herbert to comment on the vitamin C story. (Nor is it "accidental" that this particular "expert" was called on. Dr. Herbert, and his committee of self-appointed medical watchdogs against "health fraud," keep peppering journalists with their press releases, letting them know they are more than available for free "consulting" services.)

Incidentally, a few years earlier, Dr. Herbert had sounded a similar warning about another, likewise inconclusive vitamin C study, which, he said, showed that taking vitamin C supplements would interfere with vitamin B-12 absorption. That also turned out to be a false alarm, but meanwhile lots of people who desperately needed extra vitamin C were scared away.

Finally, if vitamin C is so bad for you, how come that we, and thousands of others who have been taking much more than 500 mg of it for many years, haven't dropped dead yet? To the contrary—speaking for ourselves—we are doing rather well, thank you.

In fact, we like to divide our total vitamin C intake about evenly between its common water-soluble form (ascorbic acid) and its fat-soluble one (ascorbyl palmitate), which can get into the fatty midlayer of cells and there prevent oxidative damage. This is something our friends Durk Pearson and Sandy Shaw, authors of *Life Extension,* have advocated for years.

In the end it all comes down to individual, informed judgment. Only a well-informed consumer can arrive at meaningful decisions on matters like these. In fact, the whole purpose of this book is to give you, the reader, the necessary, scientific information on which to base your decisions about a very large variety of different nutritional supplements. You will therefore have a solid, science-based body of information upon which to make up your own mind about all these matters and decide for yourself what seems right for you.

Chapter 2

How to Take Nutritional Supplements

If nutritional supplements, such as vitamins and other antioxidants, are to truly boost our immune systems, help prevent disease, and prolong life, they must be taken as part of an integrated, well-thought-out, holistic program. Only in this way can each individual micronutrient protect, support, and complement the others.

A comprehensive vitamin/antioxidant program like this must, of course, be firmly based on all the "essential" vitamins. First of all, the antioxidant vitamins C, E, and A (or its forerunner beta-carotene, from which the body manufactures its own vitamin A, as needed)* and the B-vitamins, including B-12, plus folic acid (another B-vitamin) must all be present.

*We prefer beta-carotene, because you can overdose on vitamin A. A good case can, however, be made for a small dose of vitamin A, along with beta-carotene, especially for extra cancer protection.

One reason for having all these micronutrients onboard is that each one plays a specific role in neutralizing specific free radicals. Another is that their interaction produces a synergistic effect that none of them can exert alone.

As the reader may recall, free radicals are oxygen-containing molecules that lack an electron and are therefore very unstable. They desperately try to make themselves complete by "stealing" electrons from neighboring molecules, thereby making these unstable as well. But because they contain flammable oxygen, this produces wildfire-like chain reactions, which "burn up" cell membranes and damage the genetic code in the nucleus of cells.

We are exposed to free radicals, in the first place, from the outside environment—from air pollution and certain foods, such as oils and fats that have become oxidized (something that is virtually unavoidable), or from proteins (meats) exposed to high heat by frying, grilling, and barbecuing. Free radicals are, however, also produced inside of us by our own natural metabolic processes. As one scientist quipped, "The only way to prevent free radical production in our bodies is to stop eating and breathing." We suggest a more practical solution—eat more of the right kinds of food, like vegetables, fruits, and grains, that contain free radical–scavenging vitamins and other antioxidants, then use supplements to bring antioxidant levels up to preventive and therapeutic levels.

One important thing to take into account, however, is that any individual antioxidant can, in the course of putting out the fires of free radicals, become itself consumed in the fires it is trying to extinguish. In other words, the individual *anti*oxidant may—by protecting the cells of our vital organs from free radical damage—become oxidized and turned into a *pro*-oxidant. The only way to prevent this is to have different antioxidants protect each other from getting oxidized—another good reason for using as wide a range of mutually supportive and protective antioxidants as possible.

Only by taking such a wide spectrum of nutritional supplements can we help them work together and complement one another, just as they do in nature. That, in fact, is the secret

"Vitamin E and glutathione are closely related and the two compounds exert mutually protecting properties: vitamin E prevents the oxidation of glutathione. . . . whereas glutathione (probably together with vitamin C) plays an important role in the regeneration of oxidized vitamin E."

Costaglio, C. and E. Rinaldi, "Vitamin E and Red Blood Cell Glutathione," in *CRC Handbook of Free Radicals and Antioxidants in Biomedicine.* Boca Raton, FLA: CRC Press, 1989.

behind all the studies showing that people who consume plenty of fruits and vegetables get cancer and other diseases less often than those who do not. The lesson is that by allowing nature to teach us how to use vitamins and other micronutrients holistically—that is, by taking them in combination, the way they occur in plants, fruits, and grains—can we expect to derive optimal health benefits from them.

On the other hand, it is not a good idea to take "one-a-day" multivitamins, as millions of people do, having been led by clever advertising to expect miraculous health benefits. Sure, multivitamins offer various combinations of vitamins and minerals. The trouble is that it is technically impossible to cram large enough dosages of all these vitamins, minerals, and other components into one single pill or capsule to do much good. The most these "one-a-day" pills can reasonably be expected to accomplish is to prevent vitamin or mineral deficiencies. Admittedly, that's a worthwhile goal. But we are talking here about using vitamins and other antioxidants to prevent disease and thereby extend our productive life span, which requires larger doses, such as are, to the best of our knowledge, available only from certain mail-order companies.*

*Our preferred multivitamin mail-order products are (in alphabetical order), 1) "Extend Core" (Vitamin Research Products, 1-800-877-2447); 2) "Life Extension Mix" (Life Extension Foundation, 1-800-544-4440); 3) "Performance Packs" and "Glutathione Health Packs" (Health Maintenance Programs, 1-800-DOCTOR-D). Ask for their catalogs.

> "It is reasonable to expect on the basis of present data that a judicious selection of diets and antioxidant supplements will increase the healthy, active life span by 5–10 years."
>
> Denham Harman, M.D., Department of Medicine and Biochemistry, University of Nebraska, College of Medicine. In *Molecular and Cellular Biochemistry,* 1988, 84:155–161.

Furthermore, vitamins taken only once a day cannot provide round-the-clock free radical protection, which is essential in preventing disease and extending life. Most vitamins and other antioxidants are water-soluble and hence eliminated within three to four hours. They must therefore be taken in divided doses—ideally, three times a day—to maintain the necessary levels in blood and tissues. (Cynics use this fact to disparage high-dose vitamin-taking as doing nothing but producing "expensive urine.") The kidneys, bladder, and intestines, though, are precisely where we need maximal antioxidant protection against mutagenic free radicals and environmental toxins.

A truly comprehensive vitamin/antioxidant program should also include a number of perhaps less popular but no less important micronutrients, such as DL-alpha lipoic acid, coenzyme Q-10, and L-carnitine (or acetyl-L-carnitine), all of which—aside from having their own health benefits—can also spare and regenerate other antioxidants.

Also included, of course, must be minerals like calcium, magnesium, manganese, selenium, potassium, zinc, and copper. Here, again, the question arises whether to take a multimineral pill or buy the individual minerals separately. As the reader may suspect, we prefer the latter. Multimineral pills often have too much of one thing—like iron—and too little of another.

In addition, for those over fifty, a supplement program should, in our opinon, include not only antioxidants but also certain hormones, which become rapidly depleted after this age. For women that means, first of all, estrogen/progesterone replacement therapy. For both sexes, however, complete hormone replacement therapy should also include melatonin and DHEA. But we must stress that nobody should go on a hormone replacement program without the guidance of a doctor or other health professional who is knowledgeable about such matters.

Finally, a truly holistic supplement program should also include some basic plant compounds (phytochemicals), preferably in powder form, so you can simply add them to foods, such as soups, salads, pasta sauce, or whatever. Most of them are natural antioxidants, or protect our health in other ways. They act, for instance, as immune system modulators, activating sluggish ones, or slowing-down overactive ones, as in autoimmune diseases like arthritis, chronic fatigue syndrome, multiple sclerosis, and lupus erythematosus.

Prominent among beneficial plant chemicals are the "carotenoids," like the beta-carotene that is part of our basic antioxidant program. They are found in carrots (hence the name), bell peppers, dark green, leafy vegetables, and brown-red sea vegetables (seaweeds).

A related plant chemical, lycopene (highest in tomatoes), has recently been found to protect specifically against prostate cancer, but seems to be prophylactic against other cancers as well.*

Two others, lutein and zeaxanthin (both highest in greens like kale, spinach, and broccoli), are especially protective with regard to cataracts and macular degeneration, a progressive eye disease that can lead to blindness, and for which there is otherwise no medical treatment. It is a good idea to also take the bioflavonoids quercetin and rutin, as nutritional supplements.

*For our lycopene supplement we use either Vitamin Research Products' Lycopene Beadlets (a loose powder), or their Lycopene Caps. To get enough bioflavonoids (rutin, hesperidin complex and quercetin) we use their Bioflavonoid Complex (1-800-877-2447). If you are taking the Life Extension Foundation's "Life Extension Mix," you are already getting an adequate amount of these protective plant chemicals. Nonetheless, an extra dose may be helpful, especially when fighting cancer or another serious illness.

tin is high in the white pulp of citrus fruits, but both of vonoids also occur in apples, as well as onions and other vegetables. They decrease risk of vascular disease, strengthen the capillaries, thereby reducing bruising and bleeding, and relieve the symptoms of allergies.* (It has recently also been discovered that quercetin improves the efficacy of the chemotherapy drug 5-FU, which should be of interest to oncologists and cancer patients).[1]

To get a better balance of all the bioflavonoids (and there are many!), we switch, for half of the year or so, to another type of flavonoids, called proanthocyanidins, made from grape seed extract. In test tube experiments, they have shown fifty times greater antioxidant capability than vitamin E and twenty times greater activity than vitamin C. Moreover, they can cross the blood brain barrier, so they can help prevent free radical damage.

In addition, we take curcumin, the active ingredient in the spice turmeric. Unfortunately, curcumin is hard to get in powder form, but we take it anyway—what's one more capsule to swallow!—because it has such powerful antioxidant, anti-inflammatory, and anticancer properties.†

As for the rest of the medicinal plant compounds, we think we can get enough of them from the foods in which they occur. For instance, there is genistein, found in soy beans and soy foods like tofu and tempeh, which is protective with regard to several types of cancer (although premenopausal women should go easy on soy foods because of their high estrogen content).

There is also catechin, a compound in green tea, which has proven anticancer properties. It exists also as a decaffeinated supplement, but we love the taste of good green tea, of which there exists a great variety, so one can never tire of it. Unfortunately, good green tea is not as readily available as black tea,

*Quercetin and rutin are both available in powder form from VRP (Vitamin Research Products). Rutin is also available from the Life Extension Foundation.

†Curcumin is an ancient Ayurvedic remedy, used for hundreds and maybe thousands of years in India. We get our curcumin capsules from an Indian company with the unlikely name America's Finest (1-800-350-3305).

except in urban centers like New York, Los Angeles, and San Francisco, with large Chinese and Japanese populations.*

Finally, a word about the old controversy of whether we should not get *all* our micronutrients from foods, rather than "pills." Frankly, we think this is a spurious argument, born from lack of understanding or prejudice. While we should, as much as possible, try to get the benefits of vitamins and other protective plant compounds from the foods that contain them, it is simply impossible to eat enough of them for optimal benefits. But we can, fortunately, take additional amounts of them in the form of nutritional supplements. Moreover, we consider the lesser-known plant chemicals like lycopene and curcumin, for example, just as important for our health as the better-known antioxidants, especially for cancer prevention.

There is no doubt in our minds that the judicious inclusion of all these natural compounds into our comprehensive supplement program, coupled with a sensible diet and exercise, will keep us in better health and add many happy and productive days and years to our lives. For whatever protects health in a general way, as well as lowering the risk of heart disease and cancer (our numbers one and two killers), is, by definition, also life-extending.

In the chapters that follow, we shall tell you how to use basic vitamins, antioxidants, minerals, and hormones like melatonin and DHEA—plus other often overlooked but vital biological antioxidants, anti-inflammatory compounds, and other natural remedies from nature's pharmacy.

*When in New York, we buy our green tea at the famous Chinese Ten Ren Tea and Ginseng shop, 75 Mott Street. They do mail-order business, so ask for their price list (1-800-292-2049, FAX: 212-349-2180). But brace yourself, or you'll be shocked by the prices really good green teas demand. Even the medium-grade Lung Ching and Pouchong varieties we enjoy so much cost $27.50 a pound, and the highest grade can cost up to $100 or more.

NOTES

1. Boersma, H. H., et al. Modulation of 5-fluourouracil-induced cytotoxicity by quercetin in two human colorectal cancer cell lines. *Planta Med.* Supplement Issue, 1993; 59:682.

Chapter 3

OUR BASIC ANTIOXIDANT PROGRAM

Our basic antioxidant program is simple, convenient, affordable, and yet contains plenty of the most essential vitamins and other micronutrients to give you a lot of free radical protection, even if you don't take any other supportive supplements like the ones we mentioned in the preceding chapter.

We are using, as the basis of our whole supplement program, a mail-order product called "Performance Packs" (1-800-DOCTOR-D). Excellent, alternative products are either the "Life Extension Mix" (Life Extension Foundation, 1-800-544-4440) or another combination product, "Extend Core" (Vitamin Research Products, 1-800-877-2447).

We are taking one of these little blister packs three times a day, with meals. They consist of two large yellow capsules, each containing 750 mg of ascorbic acid (vitamin C), plus all the essential B-vitamins, and 100 mcg of folic acid. The white capsule contains 100 mg of the important antioxidant glutathione, plus calcium with vitamin D-3. There is also a small, round, soft-gel capsule with 250 IU of liquid vitamin E.

Since every one of these Performance Packs gives us 1,500 mg of vitamin C, taking three Performance Packs a day would result in getting 4,500 mg of vitamin C a day—really much more than one needs, unless one is fighting a cold or has to cope with some other health emergency, such as an injury or burn, surgical trauma, or some other illness, in which case the body needs extraordinarily large amounts of vitamin C. (Persons with oxalate kidney stones, though, should *not* take vitamin C supplements.)

Normally, we therefore remove one of the yellow capsules every time we take our Performance Packs, which still leaves us with fully 2,250 mg (three times 750 mg) of this important vitamin and antioxidant. At the same time, it does not short-change us with regard to the B-vitamins (Performance Packs have much larger amounts of B-vitamins than any other such product we know of).

So, what are we doing with the extra yellow capsules with vitamin C and the B-vitamins? We collect them for possible emergencies in a separate container and store them in the refrigerator, together with the boxes of Performance Packs and all the other nutritional supplements we are taking. (You should keep *all* of your vitamins and other supplements in the refrigerator, for they are very prone to degradation by heat and light, except the minerals, which don't need refrigeration.) Then, when a lot of the yellow capsules have accumulated and there has been no emergency to use them up, there is always someone in our extended family who needs them. (Even with this give-away routine, Performance Packs are still a good bargain in terms of cost per gram, especially considering their content of the expensive antioxidant, glutathione—something that is unparalleled in the whole vitamin industry.)

On the other hand, if you opt for the Life Extension Mix of the Life Extension Foundation or the "Extend Core" product from Vitamin Research Products, you should supplement that program with at least one 250 mg capsule of glutathione per day, for instance, from Health Maintenance Programs. (See page 18 for toll-free phone numbers.)

If you should decide to take neither the Performance Packs nor the Life Extension Mix nor VPR's Extended Core but are putting your basic vitamin/antioxidant program together some other way (for instance, from individual health food store items), please use the daily dosages given below for the different vitamins as a guide:

Vitamin C (ascorbic acid)	2,000 mg
Vitamin E (DL-alpha tocopheryl acetate or succinate)	750–1,200 IU (International Units)
Beta-carotene (provitamin A)	45 mg = 75,000 IU
Glutathione	100–250 mg
B-1 (thiamine)	100–150 mg
B-2 (riboflavin)	2 mg
B-3 (as niacin or niacinamide)*	50–100 mg
B-5 (calcium pantothenate)	350–400 mg
B-6 (pyridoxine HCI)	25–50 mg
B-12 (cyanocobalamine)	600–750 mcg (microgram)
Calcium (preferably as the citrate, but carbonate acceptable)	500–750 mg
D-3 (ergocalciferol, to assist in calcium absorption)	300 IU
Folic acid	400–800 mcg†

Note: Do not leave out any of the micronutrients on the list. Each one of them plays an important role in your total program. They all work together and recycle each other, so that they are always in their fresh, bioactive form, the only form in which they can do us any good.

*In low dosages, as here suggested, niacin (rather than niacinamide) should be used, because it alone has a cholesterol-lowering effect. Higher dosages though, can produce a histamine reaction in the form of a prickly flush.

†Each Performance Pack contains 100 mcg of folic acid, so at three packs a day, we would be at least 100 mcg short of the minimum dosage recommended by the Centers for Disease Control. We are therefore taking an additional 400 mcg or 800 mcg a day from another source. If you are taking the Life Extension Mix or the Extend Core product at the recommended dosage, you don't need any additional folic acid.

Chapter 4

Are Antioxidants Compatible with Chemotherapy and Radiation Therapy?

For persons with cancer, there frequently arises the controversial question whether one can take vitamins and other antioxidants while in chemotherapy or radiation therapy.

Overwhelming scientific evidence indicates that it is not only all right but even *vital* to take antioxidants while undergoing these therapies. The problem is that many oncologists are still far behind recent research on this important point. They think that vitamins and other antioxidants are not only useless but actually do harm.

One wouldn't think that even an "alternative medicine" guru like Dr. Andrew Weil would buy into this kind of medical dogma. Ironically, however, at a conference on alternative medicine we attended, he answered a question about cancer and antioxidants by repeating the medical prejudice that people should not take antioxidants while in therapy but should do so afterward.

Eberhard challenged Dr. Weil on this, stating that other well-qualified authorities—like Dr. Charles Simone, an oncologist who has worked at the National Cancer Institute and the National Institutes of Health—were of a different opinion.* To his credit, Dr. Weil admitted that perhaps he ought to look further into this matter.

Since this is, however, an issue of great concern to so many people, we thought it best to reproduce here, by permission, the text of a statement Dr. Simone has prepared for his own patients:

Do Vitamins or Minerals Interfere with Chemotherapy or Radiation Therapy?

> This is a question I am asked frequently by patients because their oncologists, ignorant of the subject, say not to take them during treament. Many studies have been done to address this. The early studies were done at the National Cancer Institute with an antioxidant called N-acetylcysteine (NAC).† They showed that it had a protective effect on the heart for patients receiving a chemotherapeutic drug called adriamycin, which is toxic to the heart. The heart was protected and there was no interference in the tumor-killing performance of adriamycin.[1]
>
> Many cellular studies[2] and animal studies[3] demonstrate that vitamins A, E, and C, as well as beta-carotene and selenium, all protect against the toxicity of adriamycin while at the same time actually enhancing its cancer-killing effects.

*The Simone Protective Cancer Center is located at 123 Franklin Corner Road, Lawrenceville, NJ 08648; 609-896-2646.

†Instead of N-acetylcysteine (NAC), which is a good but synthetic drug, we prefer its natural equivalent, glutathione.

Animal Studies: Studies using beta-carotene and other retinoids, vitamin C, and vitamin K, [all] show that normal tissue tolerance was improved in animals undergoing both chemotherapy and radiotherapy, and tumors regressed.[4]

Vitamin E produced similar findings: no interference with the killing of tumors by either radiation or chemotherapy in animals given concomitant vitamin E.[5] Animals given both beta-carotene and vitamin A with radiation and chemotherapy had more tumor killing than with chemotherapy and radiation alone, normal tissues were more protected, and there was a longer period of time without tumor recurrence.[6]

Selenium and cysteine also heighten tumor killing by chemotherapy and radiation while, at the same time, protecting normal tissue.[7]

Cellular Studies: All cellular studies using vitamins (C, A, K, E, D, beta-carotene, B-6, B-12), minerals (selenium), and cysteine with chemotherapy and radiation have shown the same effect: increased tumor killing and increased protection of the normal tissues.[8]

Human Studies: Many human studies [about this matter] have been done. Vitamin E reduced the toxicity without affecting the cancer-killing of 13-cis-retinoic acid in the treatment of patients with head and neck, skin, and lung cancers.[9] At 1,600 IU of vitamin E per day, hair loss in patients receiving chemotherapy was reduced from the expected 30–90%.[10] Treating 190 head and neck cancer patients with vitamin A, 5-FU, and radiation resulted in more than expected tumor killing while preserving normal tissue.[11] And vitamin A combined with chemotherapy for postmenopausal patients with metastatic breast cancers significantly increased the complete response rate.[12] In thirteen patients with different cancers receiving different chemotherapies, vitamin K decreased tumor resistance.[13] Vitamin B-6 at 300 mg per day decreased radiation therapy toxicity.[14]

Twenty patients receiving chemotherapy with vitamins A, C, and E had a greater response rate.[15] Studies show that WR-2721, an antioxidant, protects against the harmful side effects of chemotherapy and radiation without the loss of antitumor activity.[16]

An *increase in survival* for cancer patients, which is uncommon with any treatment, has been shown *using antioxidants* combined with chemotherapy or radiation. Eleven patients who were given beta-carotene and canthaxanthin while undergoing surgery, chemotherapy, and radiation lived longer with an increase in disease-free interval.[17] And antioxidant treatment with chemotherapy and radiation prolonged survival for patients with small-cell lung cancer compared to patients who did not receive antioxidants.[18]

The effects of only one chemotherapeutic agent, methotrexate, can be reversed with folinic acid, which is an analog of the vitamin folic acid. Folic acid itself does not reverse methotrexate's effects. In order to reverse the effects of methotrexate, folinic acid has to be given in high doses. It cannot be obtained over the counter; it must be prescribed.

All studies show that vitamins and minerals do not interfere with the antitumor effects of chemotherapy or radiation therapy. In fact, on the contrary, some vitamins and minerals used in conjunction with chemotherapy and/or radiation therapy have been shown to protect normal tissue and potentiate the destruction of cancer cells.[19]

Having cited no fewer than forty-seven scientific sources on the subject of vitamins and other nutritional supplements with respect to chemotherapy and radiation therapy, as well as drawing on his own clinical observations, Dr. Simone concludes:

Vitamins and minerals do not interfere with the antitumor effects of chemotherapy or radiation therapy. In fact, on

> the contrary, some vitamins and minerals used in conjunction with chemotherapy and/or radiation therapy have been shown to protect normal tissue and potentiate the destruction of cancer cells . . .

In light of Dr. Simone's conclusive evidence, we would not hesitate to continue our entire nutritional supplement program under these circumstances. In fact, if anything, we would rather *increase* the dosages of our antioxidants to try to offset the tremendously increased free radical damage arising from these highly toxic therapies. But it is impossible to advise others in matters like this. Nor would it be practical; most people, even if aware of the problem, would simply be told by their doctors not to do so and would be best off just to comply, or look for a doctor who feels differently.

The medical controversy about the use of antioxidants during chemotherapy or radiation therapy is especially pronounced with regard to the key antioxidant, glutathione. We shall discuss the scientific pros and cons with regard to this issue in Chapter 9.

NOTES

1. Carlson, R. Reducing the cardiotoxicity of the anthracyclines. *Oncology,* 1992; 6(6): 96–108.
2. Taper, H., et al. Potentiation of chemotherapy in vivo in an ascitic mouse liver tumor, and growth inhibition in vitro in 3 lines of human tumors by combines vitamin C and K3 treatment. European Assn. Cancer Res., Tenth Biennial Meeting, Sept. 1989, Galway, Ireland.

   Shimpo, et. al. Ascorbic acid and adriamycin toxicity. *Am. J. Clin. Nutr.,* 1991; 54:1298S–1301S.

   Ripoll, E. A., et al. Vitamin E enhances the chemotherapeutic effects of adriamycin on human prostatic carcinoma cells in vitro. *J. Urol.,* 1986; 136(2):529–31.

   Pieters, R., et al. Cytotoxic effects of vitamin A in combination with vincristine, daunorubicin and 6-thioguanine upon cells from lympholastic leukemia patients. *Jap. J. Cancer Res.,* 1991; 82(9):1051–5.
3. Van Vleet, et al. *Cancer Treat. Reports,* 1980; 64:315.

   Singal, P. K., et al. *Molecular and cellular Biol.,* 1988; 84–163.

Wang, Y. M., et al. Effect of vitamin E against adriamycin-induced toxicity in rabbits. *Cancer Res.,* 1980; 40:1022–27.

Milei, J., et al. Amelioration of adriamycin-induced cardiotoxicity in rabbits by vitamins E and A. *Am. Heart J.,* 1986; 111:95.

Svingen, B., et al. Protection against adriamycin-induced skin necrosis in the rat by dimethyl sulfoxide and alpha-tocopherol. *Cancer Res.,* 1981; 41:3395–99.

4. Taper, H., et al. *op. cit.,* 72.

Mills. Retinoids and cancer. *Soc. R. Radiotherap. Cong.,* May 1982.

Okunieff, P. Interactions between ascorbic acid and radiation of bone marrow, skin, and tumor. *Am. J. Clin. Nutr.,* 1991; 54:1281S–83S.

Taper, H., et al. Non-toxic potentiation of cancer chemotherapy by combined C and K3 vitamin. *Int. J. Cancer,* 1987; 40:575–79.

Crary, E. J., et al. *Medical Hypothesis,* 1984; 13:77.

Sprince, H., et al. *Agents and Actions,* 1975; 5(2):164.

Poydock, E. *IRCS Medical Science,* 1984; 12:813.

5. Holm, et al., 1982. Tocopherol in tumor irradiation and chemotherapy studies in the rat. Linderstrom-Lang Conference: Selenium, vit. E and glutathion-peroxidase. Icelandic Biochem. Soc., June 25, 1982; 118.

Kagerud, A., et al. Effect of tocopherol in irradiation of artificially hypoxic rat tumors. 2nd Rome Internatl. Symposium, Sept. 1980: Biological basis and clinical implications; 3–9.

Kagerud, A., and Peterson. Tocopherol in tumor irradiation. *Anticancer Res.,* 1981; 1:35–38.

6. Shen, et al. Antitumor activity of radiation and vitamin A used in combination on Lewis lung carcinoma. 31st Annual Meeting Rad. Res. Soc., San Antonio, TX, Feb. 27, 1983; 145.

Seifter, et al. C3HBA tumor therapy with radiation, beta-carotene and vitamin A. A two year follow up. *Fed. Proc.* 1983; 42:768.

7. Williamson, J. M., et al. Intracellular cysteine delivery system that protects against toxicity by promoting glutathione synthesis. *Proc. Natl. Acad. Sci.,* 1982; 79:6246–49.

Ohkawa, K., et al. The effects of co-administration of selenium and cis-platin on cis-plating induced toxicity and antitumour activity. *Br. J. Cancer,* 1988; 58:38–41.

8. Waxman, S., et al. The enhancement of 5-FU antimetabolic activity by leucovorin, menadione, and alpha-tocopherol. *Eur. J. Cancer Clin. Oncol.,* 1982; 18(7):685–92.

Watrach, A. M., et al. Inhibition of human breast cancer cells. *Cancer Letters*, 1984; 25: 41–47.

DeLoecker, W., et al. Effects of vitamin C and vitamin K3 treatment on human tumor cell growth in vitro. Synergism with combined chemotherapy action. *Anticancer Res.*, 1993; 13(1):103–106.

Ferrero, D., et al. Self-renewal inhibition of acute myeloid leukemia clonogenic cells by biological inducers of differentiation. *Leukemia,* 1992; 6(2):100–106.

Schwartz, J. L., et al. Beta-carotene and/or vitamin E as modulators of alkylating agents in SCC-25 human squamous carcinoma cells. *Cand. Chemo. &. Pharma.*, 1992; 29(3):207–13.

Zhang, L., et al. Induction by bufalin on human leukemia cells HL60 . . . and synergistic effect in combination with other inducers. *Cancer Res.*, 52(17):4634–41.

Hofali and Waage. Effect of pyridoxine on tumor necrosis factor activities in vitro. *Biotherapy,* 1992; 5(4):285–90.

Petrini, et al. Synergistic effects of interferon and D3. *Haematologica,* 1991; 76(6):467–71.

Saunders, et al. Inhibition of ovarian carcinoma cells by taxol combined with vitamin D and adriamycin. *Proc. Ann. Meet. Am. Assn. Cancer Res.*, 1992; 33:A2641.

Ermens, A. A., et al. Enhanced effect of MTX and 5FU on folate metabolism of leukemic cells by B12. *Proc. Ann. Meet. Am. Assn. Cancer Res.*, 1987; 28:275.

9. Dimery, et al. Reduction in toxicity of high-dose cis-retinoic acid with vitamin E. *Proc. Ann. Meet. Am. Soc. Clin. Oncol.*, 1992; 11:A399.
10. Wood, L. A. *NEJM*, Apr. 18, 1985.
11. Komyjama, et al. Synergistic combination of 5FU, vitamin A, and cobalt radiation for head and neck cancer. *Auris, Nasus, Laryn.*, 1985; 12S2: S239–43.
12. Israel, L., et al. Vitamin A augments the effects of chemotherapy in metastatic breast cancers after menopause. Randomized trial in 100 patients. *Annales De Medecina Interna,* 1985; 135(7):551–54.
13. Nagourney, et al. Menadiol with chemotherapies: feasibility for resistance modification. *Proc. Meet. Am. Soc. Clin. Oncol.*, 1987; 6:A132.
14. Ladner, H. L., et al. In *Vitamins and Cancer,* F. L. Meyskens, ed. Clifton, NJ: Humana Press, 1986; 429.
15. Sakamoto, A., et al. In *Modulation and Mediation of Cancer by Vitamins,* Basel: Karger, 1983; 330.
16. Schein, P. Results of chemotherapy and radiation therapy protection trials with WR-2721. *Cancer Investigation,* 1992; 10(1):24–26.
17. Santamaria, B., et al. First clinical case report (1980–88) of cancer

chemoprevention with beta carotene plus canthaxanthin supplemented to patients after radical treatment. In *Nutrition, Growth and Cancer.* G. R. T. Tryfiates and K. N. Prasad, eds. NY: Alan R. Liss, 1988.

18. Jaakkola, et al. Treatment with antioxidant and other nutrients in combination with chemotherapy and irradiation in patients with small cell lung cancer. *Anticancer Res.,* May–June 1992; 12(3): 599–606.
19. Henriksson, et al. Interaction between cytostatics and nutrients. *Med. Oncol. Tumor Pharmacother.,* 1991; 8(2):79–86.

Part Two

Our Additional Supplement Program

Chapter 5

Vitamin E

In addition to our basic vitamin/antioxidant program, we recommend a number of other important supplements. The list is rather large; in fact, it may be overwhelming to the reader not accustomed to taking multiple supplements. But we do not mean that everybody should take all of these supplements. Rather, we suggest that you look at the following description of the various supplements as you would look at a buffet lunch or smorgasbord—picking and choosing those nutrients that seem to be most appropriate and important in terms of your particular health needs—not to mention economic constraints!

We are both taking 400 IU of additional liquid vitamin E, in the morning and in the evening, giving us—together with the 750 IU from our basic program—a total of 1,500 IU per day. (If you are not using the Performance Packs for your base program, aim for a dosage of 800–1,200 IU).

In our particular case, our first soft-gel capsule of liquid vitamin E (250 IU), taken after breakfast, together with DHEA (and Phyllis's estrogen/progesterone), is to make the hormones better absorbable. In addition, it is to prevent oxidation of the highly unsaturated flaxseed and borage oils we are taking at the same time. (See the chapters on flaxseed and borage oils.) It can also be expected to prevent the formation of oxidation products from the DHEA, which might otherwise have a toxic effect on the liver.

The heart-protective effect of vitamin E is well known and abundantly documented. Less well known is the fact that vitamin E supplementation protects the fatty midlayer of cell membranes and other fatty body tissue from free radical attack and "peroxidation" (rancidity).[1] As one scientist put it, "Vitamin (E) is the main free radical trap and antioxidant in [cell] membranes."[2]

This protective effect against oxidation (or, more accurately, peroxidation) of body fats extends not only to fats in tissue, but also to circulating fats in the blood stream. As such, it helps prevent the peroxidation of cholesterol, as well as platelet aggregation in arteries; the main causes of heart attack and stroke.

Vitamin E also protects lung tissue from damage by environmental pollutants, such as ozone and nitrogen dioxide in smog.[3] It is, furthermore, a "potent inhibitor of nitrosamine formation."[4] Nitrosamines are powerful carcinogens that occur, for various reasons, in foods (for instance, when foods are cooked in a gas oven, which is the reason why we much prefer using electric stoves).

All of this suggests that vitamin E (like vitamin C) is protective not only with regard to heart disease, but also cancer. There are some animal studies to this effect, for instance, with regard to colon and mammary (breast) tumors in rats. Some scientists have therefore concluded that "vitamin E, together with vitamin A and C may be used in cancer prevention," and that "establishing optimal levels of antioxidants such as vitamin E should be an important priority in cancer research."[5]

NOTES

1. Hennekens, C. H., M. J. Stampfer, and W. Willet. Micronutrients and cancer chemoprevention, in *Cancer Detection and Prevention*, 1984; 7:147–58.
2. Ames, B. N. Dietary carcinogens and anticarcinogens. *Science*, 1983; 221: 1256–64.
3. Ibid., n. 83.
4. Ibid., n. 85.
5. Colston, K., M. J. Colston, and D. Feldman. 1.25-dihydrovitamin D-3 and malignant melanoma: the presence of receptor and inhibition of cell growth in culture. *Endocrinology*, 1981; 108: 1083–86.

Chapter 6

Beta-Carotene and Other Carotenoids

We have, for many years, taken at least 45 mg (75,000 IU) of beta-carotene a day. (It used to be part of the Performance Packs, but was replaced by a vitamin E capsule, so we had to look for beta-carotene elsewhere.) Since then we have used a product that gives us only about a third of the beta-carotene we were getting before, but supplies other types of carotenes like alpha carotene, gamma carotene, lycopene,* and the xanthophylls (lutein, cryptoxanthin, and zeaxanthin).

*Even when taking CAROTEAM (Vitamin Research Products, 1-800-877-2447), the product with multiple carotenes, which contains some lycopene, Eberhard is still taking some additional lycopene for extra precaution against prostate cancer (see Chapter 7).

When unable to get this product, we simply go back to using straight beta-carotene caps.*

Why have we always taken beta-carotene? The main reasons, in a nutshell, are because beta-carotene:

- enables the body to produce its own vitamin A, but only the amount it needs, without danger of overdosing
- has proven anticancer effects
- is antiatherosclerotic
- provides radiation protection (acts as an internal "sunscreen")
- protects normal, healthy tissue during radiation therapy
- protects vision (together with vitamin C and glutathione) against cataracts and macular degeneration

As already said, you cannot overdose on beta-carotene. The worst thing that can happen if you take a lot of it is that your skin may take on a yellowish hue (which can also happen if you drink lots of carrot juice). No harm in any of that; rather, it provides some internal UV sun protection. Yet, some people have made that, too, sound like some kind of dangerous side effect.

More recently, though, a serious beta-carotene scare swept the country. In 1994, a team of Finnish researchers, and in 1996, a team of U.S. researchers, reported on their studies designed to test whether beta-carotene would protect heavy smokers from cancer. To everyone's consternation, they found that not only did beta-carotene not protect smokers against cancer, it seemed to make matters worse, increasing cancer rates among smokers who took it. Even the addition of a small amount of vitamin E did not seem to help. (It turned out, in the end, that the amount of vitamin E was not nearly enough to keep the beta-carotene

*You can find beta-carotene in any health food store, but we prefer the one manufactured by the giant chemical firm, Hoffman-LaRoche, used in the beta-carotene caps from the Life Extension Foundation (1-800-544-4440).

in its cancer-protective, antioxidant state. But in the excitement of the new, scary findings, nobody paid any attention to such fine points.)

Neither did many people remember previous epidemiological studies, which clearly showed that people who consume a lot of beta-carotene–rich fruits and vegetables have less cancer and other diseases than those who don't. (Carotenoids in fruits and vegetables other than beta-carotene got most of the credit for these beneficial effects, and the whole thing was given a profood, antisupplement spin.)

Newspaper headlines across the country screamed alarmist messages: "Beta Carotene Found to Increase Cancer Risk!" Thousands of people stopped taking beta-carotene. Even some vitamin manufacturers removed beta-carotene from their multiple-vitamin formulations. Supplement-haters had a field day.

But slowly, over the following months, other scientists started taking a closer look at those perplexing beta-carotene studies. They pointed out that in heavy smokers—whose physiological status, by the way, differs greatly from that of nonsmokers—beta-carotene may indeed work as a pro-oxidant, rather than an antioxidant. In that case, it would obviously make matters worse. Also, it transpired that many of the people in the Finnish study were not only heavy smokers—they were also heavy drinkers. That, again, was bound to affect the study results.

Other scientists have since pointed out the problems with testing the effectiveness of single vitamins and other antioxidants like beta-carotene. They have shown, as do we, that you have to use a broad spectrum of vitamins and other antioxidants to achieve a protective effect, since all of these substances depend on one another for their own recycling and to keep them in their fresh, antioxidant state. That's exactly why studies comparing people who consume a lot of fruits and vegetables—all of which contain many different antioxidants—with those who don't always show that those who do get fewer chronic illnesses, have lower cancer rates, and live longer.

Meanwhile, the much-maligned beta-carotene has almost regained the ground it lost after the two confounding studies with smokers. Ironically, beta-carotene's rehabilitation came in a roundabout way: concern about Procter & Gamble's fat substitute, Olestra! It was discovered that by munching Olestra-deep-fried potato chips not only could people get gastrointestinal upsets; the body was also deprived of fat-soluble beta-carotene and other carotenoids. In that connection, the Department of Health and Human Services, the National Cancer Institute, and the World Cancer Research Fund all rediscovered that carotenoids play a "potentially beneficial role in reducing the risk for cancer and certain other chronic diseases."* Consequently, carotenoids, including beta-carotene, are now routinely added to Olestra.

In that connection, the FDA acknowledged, with the double-talk characteristic of bureaucracies, that "carotenoids have not been proven with certainty to provide human health benefits, but numerous biochemical, clinical and epidemiologic studies indicate that carotenoids are likely to protect against several cancers."

The whole hubbub about beta-carotene just shows how dangerous it is to let ourselves be thrown off course by sensationalist press reports about the alleged dangers of this or that vitamin or supplement. In the case of vitamin C and beta-carotene, there had been literally hundreds of carefully conducted studies that had unequivocally shown many health benefits for these antioxidants. Nonetheless, when the overblown reports about their alleged dangers exploded in the media, all the previous evidence to the contrary seemed, at least temporarily, forgotten. Rather than protecting people, the unnecessary scare actually turned out to do a lot of harm.

*Marian Burros, "Fat Substitute May Cause Disease, a Top Researcher Says," *The New York Times*, 11 June 1998.

Chapter 7

Lycopene: The Prostate Saver

While most vitamins and other antioxidants are water-soluble, lycopene—just like its sister carotenoid, beta-carotene—is fat-soluble. This particular property alone gives it special importance, since it can protect us where water-soluble vitamins cannot. But as important as that is in its own right, lycopene shares this feature with all the other carotenoids (not to mention vitamin E, melatonin, and the still little-known and underappreciated lipoic acid, which is both water-soluble and fat-soluble).

Lycopene does play a unique role, though, in that it is the only antioxidant able to protect men from every man's biggest health concern—prostate cancer.

The question then is: Where does this "prostate saver" and—as we shall see, general anticancer compound—come from, and how can we make sure to get enough of it?

Oddly enough, we have the Aztec emperor Montezuma to thank for the fact that we even know about lycopene. He offered, as a token of hospitality, some scarce and precious tomatoes to the notorious Spanish conquistador Hernando Cortés. The latter's idea of returning the favor was to slaughter Montezuma, along with thousands of his people, and to rule Mexico from 1529 to 1531.

In the decades that followed, the Spanish, who had become fond of tomatoes, started cultivating this New World delicacy and also planted them in what later became Texas, New Mexico, Arizona, and California.

It took surprisingly little time for tomatoes to get to Europe, where they are mentioned in Italian documents as early as 1554. So popular, in fact, did tomatoes remain in Italy that, a few years ago, epidemiologists began wondering whether the low rate of prostate cancer among Italian men might not have something to do with their tomato-rich "Mediterranean diet."

It turned out, they were right: the low rate does indeed result from the fact that Italians traditionally consume tomatoes, in one form or another, almost daily. And the compound in tomatoes responsible for this protective effect is none other than lycopene (which, incidentally, also gives them their red color).[1]

Why Does Lycopene Have Anticancer Effects?

Lycopene—and *only* lycopene among all carotenoids, including beta-carotene—has this prostate-saving effect. Scientists, of course, wondered why this is so. They found that as an antioxidant, lycopene is able to best quench the highly dangerous oxygen free radical called singlet oxygen. Other antioxidants can also scavenge singlet oxygen radicals, but not in fatty tissue, as lycopene does. And the prostate, like all glands (including the testes and ovaries), is a "fatty" organ.[2]

Lycopene has also been shown to be highly protective against the hydrogen peroxide generated by our own metabolism, which is able to generate hydroxyl radicals that can damage our genetic-code-carrying DNA.[3] Lycopene is twice as active as beta-carotene in limiting this type of damage. So there is ample reason for lycopene's especially protective effect with regard to prostate cancer.

Lycopene and Various Other Cancer Risks

Lycopene is also a powerful inhibitor of endometrial, breast, and lung cancer cell proliferation (much more so than beta-carotene and the lesser-known but equally important alpha-carotene).[4]

Lycopene has even been shown to inhibit growth and development of malignant brain cells.[5]

Furthermore, a carefully designed study in mice with a tendency to develop spontaneous breast cancer showed that consistent intake of lycopene "markedly delayed and reduced tumor growth."[6]

Another equally well-designed and well-conducted study in women with early-stage cervical cancer, and a matched group of healthy women as controls, showed that lycopene (but no other carotenoid) had a strong inhibiting effect on this dangerous cancer.[7]

Lycopene and Digestive Tract Cancer

Dr. Helga Gerster,[8] director of the Vitamin Research Department, F. Hoffmann-La Roche Ltd., in Basel, Switzerland, who has done a comprehensive survey of the potential role of lycopene in human health, tells of "one of the oldest but best conducted studies involving lycopene-containing foods." It looked at dietary intakes and lifestyle factors in Iranian males with regard to esophageal cancer, and showed a "significant 40% risk reduction" from as little as one tomato-rich meal a week.[9]

Other population studies cited by Dr. Gerster showed high lycopene intake to result in "reduced cancer risk at all sites, but especially so for cancers of the stomach, colon and rectum."[10]

Lycopene and Prostate Cancer

A study involving 14,000 Seventh-Day Adventist men found that tomato consumption of five or more servings per week resulted in a "significantly decreased [prostate cancer] risk."[11]

These findings were confirmed in a more recent study, which showed that lycopene intake from tomato sauce, followed by tomatoes and pizza (but not overall intake of fruit and vegetables) was responsible for reduced prostate cancer risk.[12] Interestingly, unprocessed tomato juice showed no protective effect, although it is known from other studies that canned or bottled tomato juice, having undergone heating during processing, does have a protective effect.

How to Get the Most Lycopene from Foods

Lycopene is unique also in that—in contrast to vitamins and all other nutrients from plants—it is most active and protective when derived from cooked rather than raw tomatoes. The problem is that lycopene from raw tomatoes is not well absorbed into the body. In other words, tomatoes have to be subjected to heat to break down the cell walls and release the lycopene out of the matrix of fiber and proteins that otherwise holds it in. That may account for the fact that tomato sauce contains up to five times as much available lycopene as fresh tomatoes.

Since lycopene, as mentioned earlier, is fat-soluble, it aids absorption if tomato sauce contains some kind of fat. Commercial tomato sauce sometimes already contains some vegetable oil. But when preparing your own tomato sauce from fresh or canned tomatoes, it is advisable to add a little oil (preferably cold pressed virgin olive oil or canola oil) to maximize the availability of lycopene.

Remember, too, that the prostate-protective effect of lycopene is dependent on how many tomato-rich meals are eaten per week. While as little as one tomato-rich food a week is somewhat protective, as shown by the Iranian study, for maximum protection a person would have to eat foods like tomato sauce, tomato paste, or tomato pizza at least two or three times a week. As for ourselves, we average no more than two such "prostate meals," as we like calling them *en famille* (the rest we make up with lycopene supplements).

NOTES

1. Gerster, H. The potential role of lycopene for human health. *J. Am. College of Nutrition,* vol. 16, no. 2, 1997; 109–26.
2. Tinkler, J. H., Truscott, W., et al. Dietary carotenoids protect human cells from damage. *J. Photochem. Photobiol. B.*, 1994; 26:283–85.
3. Lu, Y., F. Ojima, et al. A new carotenoid, hydrogen peroxide oxidation products from lycopene. *Biosci. Biochem.*, 1995; 59:2153–55.
4. Levy, J., Y. Sharoni, et al. Lycopene is a more potent inhibitor of human cancer cell proliferation than either alpha-carotene or beta-carotene. *Nutr. Cancer,* 1995; 24:257–66.
5. Wang, C. J., M. Y. Chou, and J. K. Lin. Inhibition of growth and development of the transplantable C-6 glioma cells inoculated in rats by retinoids and carotenoids. *Cancer Lett.*, 1989; 48:135–42.
6. Nagasawa, H., K. Yamamoto, et al. Effects of lycopene on spontaneous mammary tumour development in SHN virgin mice. *Anticancer Res.*, 1995; 15:1173–78.
7. VanEewyck, J., F. G. Davis, and P. E. Bowen. *Int. J. Cancer,* 1991; 48: 34–38.
8. Gerster, H. op. cit., p 116.
9. Cook-Mozaffari, P. J., B. Aramesh, et al. Oesophageal cancer studies in the Caspian Littoral of Iran: results of a case-control study." *Brit. J. Cancer,* 1979; 39:293–309.
10. Franceschi, S., E. Negri, et al. Tomatoes and risk of digestive-tract cancers. *Int. J. Cancer,* 1994; 59:181–84.
11. Mills, P. K., et al. Cohort study of diet, lifestyle, and prostate cancer in Adventist men. *Cancer,* 1989; 64:598–604.
12. Giovannucci, E., W. C. Willet, et al. Intake of carotenoids and retinol in relation to risk of prostate cancer. *J. Natl. Cancer Inst.*, 1995; 87:1767–76.

Chapter 8

Folic Acid

The minimum dose for this supplement is 400 mcg (microgram) per day, as recommended by the Centers for Disease Control in Atlanta.

We get 300 mcg a day from our three Performance Packs, a hundred micrograms short of the minimum. Since higher doses of folic acid protect against colon cancer, we simply take an additional 400 mcg capsule a day, for a total of 700 mcg.

Taking a minimum of 400 mcg of folic acid per day is advisable, since marginal deficiencies of this B-vitamin are common. Yet folic acid—or folate, as it is also called—is an important micronutrient. Without it, the body cannot break down a compound called homocysteine, which then builds up in the bloodstream, tripling one's chances of a heart attack.

What interests us even more is that it also protects against adenomas—the tumors in the colon that are the beginning of serious cancer (sarcomas), with which Eberhard has had some personal and not altogether pleasant experience.

It was found that people who develop adenomas in the colon or rectum somehow don't get enough folate. One of the main sources for it is green, leafy vegetables. (In fact, *folium* in Latin means leaf or page.) Perhaps Eberhard didn't eat enough of these vegetables during our less-nutrition-conscious life, or perhaps it was all the wonderful wine and the fabulous, rich cheeses during our "wanton" Paris years that produced a folate deficiency. (Alcohol interferes with folate absorption and the high fat content of the tasty cheeses may also have played a part in the tumor formation.)

Jane Brody, nutrition writer of *The New York Times* (with whom we do not always agree, but do in this case) cites studies showing that folate apparently protects against cancer by aiding in the production of certain chemicals that, in turn, enable our DNA to resist the action of cancer-causing genes. Ms. Brody quotes a famous cancer researcher, Edward Giovannucci, M.D., as saying that "in a study of people with ulcerative colitis who face an abnormally high risk of developing colon cancer, precancerous changes in the colon were less often found in those who take folate supplements."

Another researcher, Joel Mason, M.D., of Tufts University, is quoted as saying that folate supplements in much higher dosages (twenty times the current recommended amount) can prevent colon cancer in people with precancerous polyps. Even a mild folate deficiency in animals prone to colon cancer, Dr. Mason said, doubles their risk of malignancy.

According to the same report, "low levels of folate have also been linked to the development of cellular abnormalities that precede cancer of the cervix in women infected with a cancer-causing strain of human papilloma-virus," while those with adequate folate levels were protected. Still other studies, Ms. Brody reports, "have suggested that low levels of folate may increase the risk of cancers of the lung, esophagus and breast."[1]

NOTES

1. *The New York Times,* 1 March 1994. Science section.

Chapter 9

GLUTATHIONE

From our basic vitamin/antioxidant supplement program, we get 100 mg of glutathione, three times per day, or a total of 300 mg. That's a lot more than most people get from their dietary supplements. The reason is that glutathione (on the production of which the Japanese have a virtual monopoly) is the most expensive ingredient in any vitamin/antioxidant product. So manufacturers cannot afford to put very much of this "Japanese gold dust," as the trade calls it, into their products, if they want to stay competitive.*

We feel, however, that even 300 mg of glutathione per day is not ideal for people like us, in the upper age brackets,

*Those using the Life Extension Mix or Extend Core are also advised to take extra glutathione.

especially for Eberhard, with a cancer history. We are therefore taking at least 250 mg of additional glutathione.*

The importance of glutathione for one's health can hardly be overstated. Laboratory experiments with animals, as well as human studies, have shown that glutathione can benefit us the following ways:

- offers protection against radiation
- binds to toxic, cancer-causing chemicals from the environment, thereby changing them into harmless substances that our bodies can eliminate
- maintains immuno-competence by protecting the white cells of the immune system against oxidative damage
- protects—together with other antioxidants—against reactive oxygen species (free radicals), as in chronic inflammation, such as rheumatoid disease and diabetes mellitus.

Our enthusiasm about glutathione, however, is not shared by everyone in the scientific community. In the face of controversy about glutathione, we therefore decided to fly to Atlanta and talk to a biochemist, Dr. Dean Jones at Emory University, one of the foremost experts on glutathione, to settle, once and for all, the question whether taking glutathione by mouth does any good.

In discussions with Dr. Jones, he pointed out that he and his co-workers at Emory University had been able to show that "orally ingested glutathione produces an immediate, measurable rise in human plasma glutathione levels."[1]

Our next question was, did he think glutathione was doing anything for people at special cancer risk, HIV positives, diabetics, and so on?

This was his reply: "In the first place, in glutathione we

*We are not aware of any manufacturer of 250 and 500 mg glutathione capsules other than Health Maintenance Programs (1-800-DOCTOR-D).

have a natural compound that is unlikely to cause serious complications, even in gram doses [that is, in megadoses of several thousand milligrams a day]. On the other hand, there is with oral glutathione a very high likelihood of it directly supporting the immune system. There is plenty of scientific evidence to that effect.[2]

"For example, cancer and HIV infection both often result in gastrointestinal distress—the malabsorption syndrome, poor appetite, and resulting, progressive weight loss—cachexis or wasting. You have a good likelihood that glutathione supplementation is going to have a beneficial effect there. At the very least, we should be able to restore normal levels of plasma glutathione by way of supplementation."

Dr. Jones stopped for a beat or two before summing it all up in a single, concise statement: "To my mind, taking glutathione is just good insurance."

We went on to ask specifically about any role for glutathione in cancer prevention or recurrence. He pointed out that there are many mutagens, or chemicals that cause mutations in the structure of our genetic blueprint-carrying DNA—things like smog, cigarette smoke, certain chemicals that may seep into the water supply, pesticide residues in food, and radon gas from the ground. The effect of such chemicals on our bodies constitutes the first step toward getting cancer. But this "initiation" stage does not necessarily lead to cancer. For a tumor to form, there must also be a "promotion" event.

"What's a typical cancer promoter?" we asked.

"There are, of course, thousands of them," Dr. Jones replied, "and they are often things nobody suspects. Take, for instance, any one of the popular, over-the-counter acne medications that contain benzoyl-peroxide. Millions of teenagers are bathing their faces with this stuff to counteract pimples—that's a typical tumor promoter.

"In the laboratory you can paint the skin of an animal, say a rat, with a carcinogen. That will be the first step in the development of cancer—the initiation—but the animal still won't develop a tumor. But when you come along a few months later, and go over that area with a promoter, like the acne medication I mentioned, bingo!—the tumor forms! In other words, both the original initiation event and the promotion event are necessary to transform a normal cell into a cancer cell.

"The good news is, glutathione is one of the most effective compounds in blocking both initiation and promotion [of cancer]. It reacts with the chemicals that cause initiation, like environmental pollutants, but it also reacts with the chemicals that cause promotion, like the acne medications I mentioned. In fact, glutathione even offers protection against such carcinogenic compounds as hydroperoxides, produced either by dietary fats, or by perfectly natural, physiological processes in our own bodies."

Finally, we asked Dr. Jones if there was any optimal dose of glutathione. He explained that there is indeed an ideal dose: for a normal, healthy adult, it is 15 mg of glutathione per kilogram of body weight. For a person weighing 120 to 130 pounds, the ideal dose would be 900 to 1,000 mg of glutathione a day (food sources give us no more than 50 to 75 mg). For a man weighing 150 to 160 pounds, it would be 1,100 to 1,200 mg—much more than most people take, if they take any glutathione at all.

Dr. Jones's experiments showed, though, that it would be counterproductive to take higher doses. In fact, plasma glutathione levels actually decrease if doses in excess of this formula are used.

Of course, people with cancer, AIDS, or diabetes can benefit from much higher doses of up to 3,000 mg a day. This is because any serious illness depletes the level of glutathione in plasma, as well as in cells and tissues, just as is the case with vitamin C.*

The only issue surrounding glutathione on which there is still some debate is whether oral glutathione from supplements

*In case of illness or injury and burns, it is advisable to increase vitamin C intake, along with glutathione.

will also get into immune system cells, especially lymphocytes—notoriously depleted by HIV—and into tissue. As researcher Neil Kaplowitz of the University of Southern California School of Medicine has pointed out recently, so much prior research has gone into these matters that "we are now poised" to definitively answer this question one way or another.[3] If, as Dr. Kaplowitz seems to suspect, the answer is positive and oral glutathione supplementation is unambiguously shown to benefit immune system cells either directly or indirectly (as a vehicle for cysteine/cystine delivery) this knowledge, he says, "can be applied to furthering the prevention and treatment of the diseases of oxidative stress, such as aging, HIV, cataract, atherosclerosis, cancer, and alcoholic liver disease."[4]

Meanwhile, however, we already have an alternative and apparently quite efficient way of getting glutathione into immune system cells and body tissue: convincing studies show that supplementing our diet with bioactive, undenatured whey protein concentrate or isolate is capable of doing so.[5]

See Chapter 40, "Whey Protein: Virtual 'Mother's Milk' for Everyone."*

Glutathione's Role in Chemotherapy and Radiation Therapy

If you are in chemotherapy or radiation therapy, you absolutely must check with your oncologist before taking glutathione. Chances are, your doctor will be dead set against your taking high doses of glutathione supplements while you undergo these treatments.

Since glutathione is especially protective against toxic substances, like those used in chemotherapy, as well as against the harmful effects of radiation therapy, most oncologists fear

*Alpha lipoic acid also increases cellular glutathione levels (see Chapter 11).

that glutathione may cancel out the effectiveness of the chemotherapy.

In actual fact, however, clinical experience seems to indicate that antioxidant supplementation, including glutathione, makes it possible for patients to tolerate higher doses of chemotherapy by reducing its nasty side effects, as oncologist, Dr. Charles Simone, points out (see Chapter 4).

As for radiation therapy, the objection to glutathione on grounds that it is known to protect against radiation also seems less than well reasoned. It is a clinically known fact that cancer cells have much higher glutathione levels than normal tissue and are, hence, much better protected. Glutathione supplementation will therefore mainly protect healthy, normal cells from radiation damage, because they are much more vulnerable to radiation than cancer cells.

At any rate, if you are in chemo- or radiation therapy, you must discuss this with your oncologist. If your doctor is definitely against taking glutathione during therapy, you have no choice but to follow that advice, or to look for another oncologist who is more open-minded and flexible.*

Speaking strictly for ourselves, if one of us were in chemotherapy and the protocol included cisplatin (Platinol), we would *insist* on taking simultaneously 500–1,000 mg of glutathione per day. The reason is that cisplatin and similar platin derivatives are so toxic to the kidneys that chemotherapy with these drugs often results in serious kidney damage.

The specific reason why glutathione does not interfere with cisplatin chemotherapy is that an enzyme needed for the intracellular transport of glutathione, which is plentiful in many vital organs like the kidneys, happens to be "scarce on the membranes of cancer cells," as a British study has pointed out.† In

*While one should always leave the reins for one's treatment in the hands of one's physician, it is also highly advisable sometimes to seek a second and even third medical opinion. The Life Extension Foundation has a Directory of Innovative Doctors, listing over one thousand physicians of various specialities (for information call 1-800-841-5433).

†The enzyme referred to is gamma-glutamyl-transferase.

> "Glutathione shields against cisplatin (Platinol) toxicity in women with ovarian cancer, with no loss of antineoplastic [anticancer] efficacy."
>
> *Congress of the European Society of Medical Oncology, 1995.*

other words, the extra glutathione from supplements cannot get into the cancer cells, but can be absorbed by the healthy cells of normal tissue, and thereby protect them.

The cited study noted that glutathione supplements "lowered the incidence of neurotoxicity . . . nephrotoxicity [kidney poisoning] . . . and anemia."* Quality-of-life assessment also showed that patients on glutathione have less nausea and vomiting (the bane of all chemotherapy, since it can cause an inability to eat or absorb food, resulting in starvation). Additional benefits were less paresthesias (tingling, pain, or numbness in hands and feet), less hair loss, and less difficulty in breathing. Glutathione supplements also reduced cognitive slippage during cisplatin therapy, such as difficulty with concentration and memory, as well as improving patients' ability to keep up with housekeeping, shopping, and so forth.

There is only one more thing to add: If there can be justified controversy whether patients should take glutathione supplements during chemo- or radiation therapy, there really can be no such controversy about the advisability of doing so after these therapies. One side effect of chemotherapy happens to be that it critically depletes one's plasma and tissue glutathione levels, just as glutathione levels in lymphocytes are depleted in HIV infection, weakening immunological defenses. Obviously, the faster and more effectively glutathione levels are restored, the better. There are many more reasons why people who have been in chemo- or radiation therapy and those who are HIV-positive should take as much glutathione as possible, whether as

*Glutathione apparently did not protect against ototoxicity (damage to hearing and the sense of balance).

nutritional supplements or in the form of undenatured whey protein concentrate,* or both.

NOTES

1. Hagen, T. M., G. T. Wierzbicka, A. H. Sillau, B. B. Bowman, and D. P. Jones. Bioavailability of dietary glutathione. Effect on plasma concentration. *Am. J. Physiol.*, 1990; 259:G524–29.

   Hagen, T. M., G. T. Wierzbicka, B. B. Bowman, T. Y. Aw, and D. P. Jones. Fate of dietary glutathione. Disposition in the gastrointestinal tract. *Am. J. Physiol.*, 1990; 259:G530–35.

   Aw, T. Y., G. T. Wierzbicka, and D. P. Jones. Oral glutathione enhances tissue glutathione in vivo. *Faseb J.*, 1990; 4:A1174.
2. Furukawa, T., S. N. Meydani, and J. B. Blumberg. Reversal of age-associated decline in immune responsiveness by dietary glutathione supplementation in mice. *Mechanisms of Aging and Development*, 1987; 38: 107–17.
3. Kaplowitz, N., et al. GSH transporters: molecular characterization and role in GSH homeostasis. *Biological Chemistry, Hoppe Seyler*, 1996; 377 (5): 267–73.
4. *Ibid.*, 267.
5. Bousnous, G., et al. The biological activity of undenatured dietary whey proteins: role of glutathione. *Clin. Invest. Med.*, 1991; vol.14:4, 296–309.

*We know of only one such product, Immunocal, that is biologically active and able to deliver glutathione to lymphocytes (1-888-462-3397).

Chapter 10

SELENIUM

We take 100–200 mcg (microgram) of this trace element a day, depending on whether we are in an area with selenium-rich or poor soils. Much of the eastern United States, for instance, has selenium-poor soils, as does Costa Rica, where we spend our winters, since Eberhard's body can no longer cope with the cold weather. So, when we are in New York, or in Costa Rica, we are taking 200 mcg of selenium.

You can supplement selenium in many different ways, since a number of companies offer this mineral in various forms. If you are, for instance, taking the Life Extension Booster Caps, you are getting three different forms of selenium, for a total of 200 mcg, 50 mcg of which is in the form of seleno-methionine, its organic and best absorbed, but not necessarily most anticarcinogenic, form.

Many people think that organic forms of selenium are superior to inorganic ones. Researchers, however, found that naturally occurring organo-selium compounds (e.g., selenomethionine) do not provide an advantage with regard to cancer protection, compared with inorganic selenium compounds, such as selenium selenate.[1]

Although selenium is technically a mineral and will also be discussed as such later, we are discussing it here first, because it is an important item in our basic supplement program. Selenium is important for many reasons. For one thing, a vital enzyme system—glutathione peroxidase—is selenium-dependent, and even marginal selenium deficiency may prevent its proper functioning. Furthermore, selenium protects against several common degenerative diseases, such as coronary artery disease, cerebrovascular disease (strokes), and degenerative joint disease (arthritis and rheumatoid arthritis). Most important to us, however, after a couple of cancer scares, is its role in boosting cellular immunity, which, as one researcher put it, "may explain in part its reported anticarcinogenicity."[2]

Recently, it has been shown that the AIDS virus slowly depletes the body of selenium—just as it does with glutathione. When the virus has used up all the selenium in an immune system cell, it breaks out in search of more, spreading the infection to other cells.

This is of special importance to those with AIDS who also have Kaposi's sarcoma, a type of cancer affecting the skin, as well as the epithelial lining of internal organs. In fact, it appears that the majority of HIV-infected people who do not show any outside symptoms (purplish patches on the skin) of Kaposi's sarcoma, nevertheless do have some internal lesions of this strange malignancy. Daily supplementation with 200 mcg of selenium, as well as with 250 to 500 mg of glutathione, three times per day, therefore seems a wise prophylactic, as well as therapeutic, strategy for anyone who is HIV-positive.

NOTES

1. El-Bayoumy, K. The role of selenium in cancer prevention. *Cancer Prevention,* March 1991; 1–15.
2. Hendler, Sheldon S. *The Doctor's Vitamin and Mineral Encyclopedia.* NY: Simon & Schuster, 1990; 184.

Chapter 11

Alpha Lipoic Acid

We are currently taking 100 mg of lipoic acid a day, after breakfast, together with our other antioxidants, DHEA, and flaxseed oil.

Alpha lipoic acid is synthesized in the body by animals as well as humans, just like glutathione (hence neither one of them is a vitamin, for we cannot synthesize vitamins). However, as in the case of glutathione, alpha lipoic acid and its reduced form, dihydrolipoic acid (DHLA), are extremely effective, broad-spectrum antioxidants and free radical scavengers. So much so, in fact, that Lester Packer, Ph.D., head of the Department of Molecular and Cell Biology, University of California at Berkeley, says that "the alpha lipoic acid/dihydrolipoic acid redox couple approaches the ideal" for any antioxidant.[1]

One of the most important features of this dual antioxidant is its ability to regenerate other essential antioxidants, such as vitamin C, vitamin E, coenzyme Q-10, and glutathione. Perhaps for this reason, laboratory experiments with both animal and human cell lines have shown that when alpha lipoic acid is added, there is an increase of 30–70% in cellular glutathione (GSH) levels. (You don't have to take dihydrolipoic acid, the reduced form of alpha lipoic acid, separately; when you take alpha lipoic acid, its reduced form is generated spontaneously in the body, so you get the benefits of both versions of this remarkable antioxidant.)

Alpha lipoic acid/dihydrolipoic acid are also proven to be extremely effective in the prevention and treatment of diabetes. There has even been dramatic improvement with lipoic acid in the painful neuropathies, typical of advanced diabetes,[2] as well as a marked reduction in cataract formation, also typical of advanced diabetes.[3] (The latter is apparantly due to the fact that lipoic acid prevents the loss of vitamin C, vitamin E, and glutathione in the lens of the eye.)[4]

Still another benefit of this twin antioxidant seems to be its ability to regenerate neurons, making it a potential therapy for such degenerative, central nervous system disorders as Alzheimer's, Parkinson's, and Lou Gehrig's diseases. It also helps prevent the memory loss that frequently accompanies advanced age.

A recent study has even found alpha lipoic acid, dissolved in propylene glycol and locally applied to the skin, to have high antioxidant activity and to protect the skin against oxidative damage.[5]

In view of these multiple benefits of lipoic acid, we can only urge readers to include it, if economically possible, in their supplement program.

NOTES

1. Dr. Lester Parker, as quoted in *Life Extension* magazine, March 1996; 4–5.
2. Packer, L. Antioxidant properties of lipoic acid and its therapeutic effects in prevention of diabetes complications and cataracts. *Annals N.Y. Acad. Sciences,* Nov. 17, 1994; 738: 257–64.
3. Spector, A. In *Human Cataract Formation* (Ciba Foundation Symposium 106). J. Nugent and J. Whelan, eds. London: Pitman, 1984; 48–64.

4. Maitra, I., E. Serbinova, H. Trischler, and L. Packer. Alpha lipoic acid prevents buthionine sulfoximine-induced cataract formation in newborn rats. *Free Radic. Biol. Med.*, April 1995; 18(4): 823–29.
5. Podda, M., et al. Kinetic study of cutaneous and subcutaneous distribution following topical application of [7, 8/14 C] rac-alpha-lipoic acid onto hairless mice. *Biochem. Pharmacol.*, 1996; 52 (4): 627–33.

Chapter 12

Coenzyme Q-10

We are both taking 30 mg of coenzyme Q-10 a day, after breakfast, along with a Performance Pack, DHEA, lipoic acid, and flaxseed oil, because CoQ-10 seems to work best in the presence of some oil.

After years of controversy in the scientific community, coenzyme Q-10 has finally made it into the famous "PDR" (*Physicians' Desk Reference*). Here is what this sacrosanct manual of the medical profession has to say:

> Coenzyme Q-10 is an essential nutrient that is a cofactor in the mitochondrial electron transport chain, the biochemical pathway in cellular respiration from which ATP and metabolic energy is derived. Since nearly all cellular functions are dependent on energy, coenzyme Q-10 is essential for the health of all human tissues and organs. The

involvment of coenzyme Q-10 as a redox carrier of the respiratory chain is well established on the basis of both reconstitution studies and kinetic evidence."
Physicians' Desk Reference, 1995 edition

As with glutathione, our bodies make some coenzyme Q-10 themselves, but not enough to offset the effects of serious illness or advanced age. Its importance lies in the fact that coenzyme Q-10 (like L-carnitine, about which more presently) is, as the PDR points out, crucial for energy production in the mitochondria of cells.*

Another reason we take coenzyme Q-10 is that it helps prevent periodontal disease, with which both of us had a painful and expensive experience some time ago.

*Mitochondria are tiny organelles in the fluid interior of cells. They are the principal sites where ATP—the universal energy storage molecule—is synthesized, without which we could not benefit from the foods we eat.

Chapter 13

L-Carnitine or Acetyl-L-Carnitine

Optimal dosage: 500 to 1,000 mg per day. It is best taken in conjunction with coenzyme Q-10 (though not necessarily at the same time), because these two nutrients complement each other in several respects.*

Taking acetyl-L-carnitine (or L-carnitine)—we shall use, from here on, only L-carnitine in reference to either one of them—is especially important in the presence of special cancer risk. With already existing cancer, however, where often weight loss is to be avoided, L-carnitine may be counterindicated. On the other hand, where losing weight is the goal, L-carnitine is one of the supplements to consider (along with chromium picolinate, chitosan, citrichrome, and other natural weight control aids).

*We take our acetyl-L-carnitine after dinner.

Like glutathione and coenzyme Q-10, L-carnitine is a naturally occurring compound, present in our cells. We also get small amounts of it from certain foods, like milk and other dairy products.

L-carnitine, like CoQ-10, is essential for efficient energy production and usage in mitochondria, the tiny energy generators inside our cells. Carnitine is, for instance, required for the transport of long-chain fatty acids across mitochondrial membranes in the liver. Without this mechanism, cells would not be able to utilize the fat from foods for energy production.

Maintenance of satisfactory cellular energy levels is particularly important for cancer survival (as it is for long-term HIV survival) and for slowing down the aging process—all of which is interconnected by complex and still poorly understood physiological mechanisms. Recently, it has also been discovered that supplementation with either L-carnitine or acetyl-L-carnitine provides significant protection against single-strand breaks of the double-stranded DNA in the nuclei of our cells.

The latest research seems to show that the much more expensive acetyl-L-carnitine is better absorbed (even by elderly persons) than just plain L-carnitine, despite the fact that the acetate portion of that compound is probably lost while traveling through the digestive system. At any rate, the vast majority of

> "Evidence that both L-carnitine and acetyl-L-carnitine can help in the repair of DNA damage in peripheral blood lymphocytes (white blood cells) suggests that these compounds can help to *prevent the age-related decline of the immune system* and, perhaps, other systems as well. DNA repair is at the very heart of all our life functions and any therapy that can aid this process is of great value."
>
> (*Life Extension Report,* a publication of the Life Extension Foundation, vol. 14, no. 8, August 1994).

L-Carnitine or Acetyl-L-Carnitine

- protects heart tissue against insufficient blood supply[1]
- improves cardiac performance[2]
- contributes to the generation of energy in heart cells[3]
- helps prevent neural cell death[4]
- helps in restoring poor mental functioning due to chronic alcoholism
- improves learning and memory (especially short-term memory) and cognitive abilities by increasing energy within neurons[5]
- counteracts depression[6]
- helps to control neural degeneration associated with diabetes or sciatica[7]
- slows down the process of nerve cell destruction in Alzheimer's and similar degenerative central nervous system diseases.[8]

the studies on which the following summary is based were actually conducted with acetyl-L-carnitine (not L-carnitine).

Summarizing Will Block's* excellent discussion of L-carnitine and its esterified form, acetyl-L-carnitine, we highlight above what appear to be its principal health benefits.

With regard to the last point—the reported improvement in the condition of Alzheimer's patients and possibly Parkinson's patients as well—the probable mechanism involved seems to be L-carnitine's interference with the usual decrease in a mitochondrial enzyme (carnitine acetyl-transferase), which is suspected of contributing greatly to these disease processes, as well as to aging itself.[9]

In addition, several studies have shown that acetyl-L-carnitine reduces the production of lipofuscin (peroxidized, "rancid" fatty deposits in cells), which increases with aging and

*Will Block is editor of *Living Longer,* a monthly newsletter on life extension and politics.

is linked to declining mental functions. This effect of acetyl-L-carnitine undoubtedly results from its antioxidant functions, particularly its ability to scavenge the superoxide radical which accounts for most of the oxidation of fats.[10]

Studies with acetyl-L-carnitine have shown that it not only has the ability to reduce accumulation of lipofuscin in the brain, but it also steps up the metabolism of the neurotransmitter acetylcholine.[11] One can probably achieve this effect also with regular L-carnitine, but since large doses of acetylcholine are needed to counteract the effects of aging on cognitive functions, equally large doses of L-carnitine are needed. It thus seems more practical to use acetyl-L-carnitine for improvement of age-related cognitive functioning. Acetyl-L-carnitine can be taken five-months-on/five-months-off. So, in the long run it is really no more expensive than regular L-carnitine, which has to be taken twelve months of the year.

NOTES

1. Paulson, D. J., M. J. Schmidt, J. Romens, and A. L. Shug. Metabolic and physiological differences between zero-flow and low-flow myocardial ischemia: effects of L-acetylcarnitine. *Basic Res. Cardiol.,* 1984; 79(5): 551–61.
2. Ruggiero, F. M., F. Cafagna, M. N. Gadaleta, and E. Quagliariello. Effect of aging and acetyl-L-carnitine on the lipid composition of rat plasma and erythrocytes. *Biochem. Biophys. Res. Commun.,* 1990; 170 (2): 621–26.
3. Paradies, G., F. M. Ruggiero, M. N. Gadaleta, and E. Quagliariello. The effect of aging and acetyl-L-carnitine on the activity of the phosphate carrier and on the phospholipid composition in rat heart mitochondria. *Biochem. Biophys. Acta Biomembr.,* 1992; 1103 (2): 324–26.
4. Manfridi, A., G. L. Forloni, E. Arrigoni-Martelli, and M. Mancia. Culture of dorsal root ganglion neurons from aged rats: effects of acetyl-L-carnitine and NGF. *Int. J. Dev. Neurosc.,* 1992; 10 (4): 321–29.
5. Petruzella, V., L. G. Baggetto, F. Penin, F. Cafagna, F. M. Ruggiero, P. Cantatore, and M. N. Gadaleta. In vivo effect of acetyl-L-carnitine on succinate oxidation, adenine nucleotide pool and lipid composition of synaptic and non-synaptic mitochondria from cerebral hemispheres of senescent rats. *Arch. Gerontol. Geriatr.,* 1992; 14 (2): 131–44.
6. Gecele, M., G. Francesetti, and A. Meluzzi. Acetyl-L-carnitine in aged subjects with major depression: clinical efficacy and effects on the circadian rhythm of cortisol. *Dementia,* 1991; 2 (6): 333–37.

7. Mezzina, C., D. De Grandis, M. Calvani, A. Marchioni, and A. Pomes. Idiopathic facial paralysis: new therapeutic prospects with acetyl-L-carnitine. *Int. J. Clin. Pharmacol. Res.*, 1992; 12 (5–6): 299–304.

   Malone, J. I., S. Lowitt, N. Corsico, and Z. Orfalian. Altered neuroexcitability in experimental diabetic neuropathy: effect of acetyl-L-carnitine administration. *Exp. Gerontol.*, 1990; 25 (2): 127–37.

   Tenconi, B., L. Donadoni, E. Germani, A. Bertelli, P. Mantegazza, A. M. DiGiulio, M. T. Ramacci, and A. Gorio. Intraspinal degenerative atrophy caused by sciatic nerve lesions prevented by acetyl-L-carnitine. *Int. J. Clin. Pharmacol. Res.*, 1992; 12 (5–6): 263–67.

8. Carta, A., and M. Calvani. Acetyl-L-carnitine: a drug able to slow the progress of Alzheimer's disease? *Ann. N.Y. Acad. Sci.*, 1991; 640: 228–32.

   Sinforiani, E., M. Iannuccelli, M. Mauri, A. Costa, P. Merlo, G. Bono, and G. Nappi. Neuropsychological changes in demented patients treated with acetyl-L-carnitine. *Int. J. Clin. Pharmacol. Res.*, 1990; 10 (1–2): 69–74.

9. *Ann. Neurol.*, 1992; 32: 583–586.

10. Geremia, E., C. Santoro, D. Baratta, M. Scalia, and G. Sichel. Antioxidant action of acetyl-L-carnitine; in vitro study. *Med. Sci. Res.*, 1988; (13): 699–700.

11. Maccari, F., A. Arseni, P. Chiodi, M. T. Ramacci, and L. Angelucci. Levels of carnitine in brain and other tissues of rats of different ages: effect of acetyl-L-carnitine administration. *Exp. Gerontol.*, 1990; 25 (2): 127–34.

Chapter 14

Aspirin

Aspirin's beneficial effects in fighting cardiovascular disease are well known, but one thing should be added: most people take far too much. One whole adult aspirin per day is excessive. We are both taking an 81 mg "baby aspirin" daily.

We do not take aspirin for protection against heart attack; our good diet and exercise, plus our vitamin C, vitamin E, and other supplements should already make us pretty safe on that score. Rather, we take a small amount of aspirin for its less well known but amply documented protection against colon cancer—even a single adult aspirin, taken once a week, can make a big difference. (Eberhard wishes he had known about this simple, preventive trick long ago. He might never have had to have a—gratefully "only" premalignant—tumor cut out of his colon.)

There is also aspirin's alleged effectiveness as an immune-booster. While this has been subjectively observed in some cases of HIV infection,[1] some scientists say that it has not yet been sufficiently researched. On the other hand, Dr. Sheldon Hendler, a medical researcher and author of several books on antioxidants, points out that "aspirin can boost production of interferon and interleukin-2," both of which are known immune-defenses.[2]

NOTES

1. James, J. S. Aspirin and AIDS. *AIDS Treatment News,* 17 August 1990; 109: 1–5.
2. Hendler, Sheldon S. *The Doctor's Vitamin and Mineral Encyclopedia.* NY: Simon & Schuster, 1990.

Part Three

Our Mineral Supplements

Chapter 15

VITAL FACTS ABOUT MINERALS

If you are now using or going to use the Life Extension Foundation's "Life Extension Mix" (1-800-544-4440), you need not worry about adding minerals from somewhere else; they're already in your mix. In our own case, though—our basic vitamin/antioxidant program consists of the Performance Packs from Health Maintenance Programs—we have to add our own minerals.*

Why are we putting up with this inconvenience? Not because we are gluttons for punishment, to be sure. It's just that, as health professionals, we want to keep our basic supplement

*We get our minerals mostly from Vitamin Research Products (1-800-877-2447). Again, if you are using either VRP's Extend Core or the Life Extension Mix, you do not need additional minerals.

program as "basic" as possible. That way, we have an absolutely free hand to add to it whatever we think we need most.

Some of you may want to do the same; for others it may be more practical to get just about everything you basically need in one single product, and have very little to add. It's really just a matter of personal preference.

In either case, you will want to know what minerals are good for, in general, and what different minerals are good for, in particular.

Starting with the more general function of minerals in human nutrition, we know that minerals are vital for

- the proper functioning of a number of enzymes
- the absorption of nutrients from the gastrointestinal tract and the uptake of nutrients by cells
- the normal functioning of the nervous system. (Mineral deficiency can lead to irritability, reduced attention span, fatigue, memory impairment, and depression)

With this general understanding about the function of minerals, we can now take a look at what each one of a select list of essential minerals can do for our health and what scientists consider ideal dosages when taken as supplements.

Selenium 100–200 mcg/day (a mixture of organic and inorganic selenium [e.g., sodium selenate] preferred).

Magnesium 170 mg/day (citrate preferred).*

Boron 3 mg/day (from chelated citrate, aspartate, or glycinate preferred, as, for instance, in TwinLab's TriBoron).

Potassium 100 mg/day (citrate or aspartate preferred).

*We like a product from Vitamin Research Products, Inc., called MPA-Magnesium/Potassium Aspartate, which combines 100 mg of magnesium with 90 mg of potassium.

Zinc 30 mg/day (zinc methionate preferred, but other forms acceptable).

Copper 2 mg/day (as, for instance, copper salycilate).

Iron 10 mg/day, but only in case of diagnosed iron-deficiency (preferably from products using non-heme iron, derived from other than meat sources).*

Manganese 10 mg/day (from chelated manganese gluconate preferred).

*Floradix Liquid Iron Formula is one, among several nonconstipating, vegetarian souces of non-heme iron, available in many health food stores, or direct from the company (1-800-446-2120).

Chapter 16

Selenium

Keep in mind that for both cancer and heart protection, selenium works best when supported by adequate vitamin E levels.[1] That isn't a problem if you follow our recommendation for taking 800–1,200 IU of vitamin E a day.

As pointed out in our discussion of vitamin E, this antioxidant protects against cancer in its own right. There is, for instance, a famous Russian study (1989), in which rats were given a powerful cancer-inducing chemical. No wonder the poor rats produced, on average, five tumors each. But when given vitamin E, they developed 37% fewer tumors.[2]

When vitamin E is, however, used together with selenium, their combined (synergistic) anticancer effect is even greater. That is because selenium acts not only as an antioxidant, but indirectly also as a potent detoxicant. It accomplishes this by means of an enzyme (glutathione peroxidase) that our bodies produce, which depends on the presence of selenium to bind to environmental carcinogens.

In addition, selenium has a marked ability to boost cellular immunity, a factor that may explain in part its reported anticarcinogenicity and protective effect with regard to cardiovascular and inflammatory joint diseases like arthritis and rheumatoid arthritis.

As pointed out earlier, it has been recently shown that the AIDS virus depletes T-cells not only of glutathione but also of selenium. When the virus has used up all the selenium and glutathione, it breaks out in search of more, spreading the infection to other immune system cells. Thus, replenishing selenium is especially important for AIDS patients (see Chapter 10).

NOTES

1. El-Bayoumy, K. The role of selenium in cancer prevention. *Cancer Prevention,* March 1991; 1–15.
2. Bespalov, V. G., et al. The effect of tocopherol and ascorbic acid on the development of experimental esophageal tumors. *Vopr. Onkol.,* 1989; 35: 1332–36.

Chapter 17

Magnesium/Boron

Magnesium works well together with calcium and boron for the prevention of osteoporosis. Aside from this bone-preserving function, magnesium is important for the synthesis of proteins and nucleic acids—our genetic code-carrying DNA and RNA.

Not much is known at this time about any anticancer effects of magnesium. What little we know, however, points to magnesium having a protective effect. Indian scientists found, for instance, that when rats were treated with a cancer-inducing chemical and then given magnesium, their tumor rate fell 58%.[1]

Other animal studies have shown that animals fed a magnesium-deficient diet have a higher cancer rate. Conversely, if animals are given a high magnesium diet, there is a preventive effect. Scientists believe that magnesium in cell membranes may protect against the mutagenic changes in cells that are the first step toward the development of cancer.[2]

Magnesium is also necessary for the metabolism of glucose, which, in turn, drives the production of cellular energy and contributes to such vital functions as our heartbeat. All of this is important not only for supplementing sports and exercise, but also for the treatment of ventricular heart dysrhythmias. Also, essential hypertension has been reduced with magnesium supplementation.

Boron complements magnesium and calcium, especially in the prevention of osteoporosis (2.5–3mg is a reasonable dose). It is also important for those engaging in strenuous sports and exercise. A study in which male body builders were supplemented with 2.5 mg of boron, in addition to magnesium, had increased plasma testosterone levels, lean body mass and strength.[3]

NOTES

1. Ramesha, A., et al. Chemoprevention of 7, 12–demethylbenz [a] anthracene-induced mammary carcinogenesis in rats by the combined actions of selenium, magnesium, ascorbic acid and retinyl acetate. *Jap. J. Cancer Res.,* 1990; 81:1239–46.
2. Blondell, J. M. The anticarcinogenic effect of magnesium. *Med. Hypothesis,* 1980; 6:863–71.
3. Vitamins and trace elements. In *Sports Nutrition.* I. Wolinsky and J. A. Driskell, eds. Boca Raton, FL: CRC Press, 1997; 208.

Chapter 18

ZINC

Zinc is one of the most vital among essential minerals. It plays a major role in the maintenance and functioning of the immune system, particularly on the cellular level. Without sufficient zinc, people and animals cannot defend themselves effectively against infections. Dr. Sheldon Hendler, author of *The Doctor's Vitamin and Mineral Encyclopedia,* cites the case of a mutant strain of cattle that has a genetic defect in the absorption of zinc. These animals have impaired cellular immunity and a reduced antibody response, making them highly susceptible to infections and premature death. But veterinary scientists discovered that zinc supplements can reverse this condition.

This has obvious implications for cancer prevention, for which a well-functioning immune system is essential. Ralph Moss, Ph.D., author of *Cancer Therapy,* cities several animal studies in which zinc was able to modify the carcinogenic effect of certain chemicals. Also, a study of human prostate tumor tissue revealed deficient concentrations of zinc and potassium, while other mineral concentrations remained normal. These findings were confirmed by a Danish study, which also found diminished zinc concentrations in prostate tumor tissue, but not in the tissue of prostates with benign (noncancerous) prostate enlargement.[1]

While zinc deficiency plays a role in the initiation of prostate cancer, zinc supplementation is vital in the adjunct therapy of prostate cancer (and possibly other cancers), for the immune system depends on adequate serum zinc levels.[2]

Zinc's main functions, however, lie elsewhere. Zinc is a component of a large number of enzymes that catalyze vital metabolic reactions. Like magnesium, it facilitates the synthesis of DNA and RNA, and thus participates in protein synthesis. This is especially important in tissues that undergo rapid turnover, such as the gastrointestinal tract, skin, and taste buds (zinc deficiency is notorious for causing loss of taste and smell).

Zinc also fosters wound healing and enhances the action of a number of hormones.

Zinc status, furthermore, is known to affect muscular performance by its involvement in aerobic metabolism. One indication of this is that intense exercise leads to lowered zinc levels. This is especially important for adolescent gymnasts, because zinc deficiency prevents normal growth hormone secretion, which, in turn, can lead to abnormalities in growth and pubertal maturation. Zinc supplementation, on the other hand, is known to improve aerobic performance and counteract these pernicious effects.[3]

Zinc is also essential for human vision. It is an important factor in the prevention of the progressive eye disease macular degeneration, which can lead to blindness. The bad news is that there is no effective medical treatment for this disease. The good news is that it has been found that zinc—in conjunction with high glutathione supplementation (1,000–1,500 mg/day), plus vitamin C, alpha lipoic acid, beta-carotene, and bioflavonoids like lutein and zeathantin—is able to slow the progression of this terrible disease and possibly halt its progression altogether.[4]

Finally, zinc lozenges, when started within the first twenty-four hours after the first symptoms of the common cold, can "significantly reduce the duration of illness . . . and [have] a clear therapeutic effect on most of the individual symptoms."[5] (Such symptomatic treatment should, however, be accompanied by the only effective antiviral treatment we know of: extract of echinacea/goldenseal.)*

Zinc and copper are antagonistic; that is, they tend to deplete each other. If you take zinc supplements, you must also take copper, and vice versa.

NOTES

1. Leake, A., et al. Subcellular distribution of zinc in the benign and malignant prostate: evidence for a direct zinc androgen interaction. *Acta Endocrinol.,* (Copenhagen) 1984; 105: 281–88.
2. Trace minerals, the central nervous system, and behavior. In Kanarek, R. B., and R. Marks-Kaufman, *Nutrition and Behavior: New Perspectives.* NY: Van Nostrand Reinhold, 1991.
3. Brun, J-F., et al. Serum zinc in highly trained adolescent gymnasts. *Biological Trace Element Research,* vol. 47, 1995; 273–78.
4. Dean Jones, Ph.D., Emory University, Department of Biochemistry. Personal communication.
5. Mossad, S. B., et al. Zinc gluconate lozenges for treating the common cold: a randomized, double-blind, placebo-controlled study. *Ann. Intern. Med.,* 1996; 125:81.

*We have had good results with Echinacea/Goldenseal extract from Gaia Herbs, Inc. (1-800-831-7780). At onset of cold or flu symptoms, take two teaspoons every two to three hours for the first twenty-four hours. Reduce the dosage gradually, depending on symptoms.

Chapter 19

Copper

We take a copper supplement (1 mg of copper salicylate) not out of concern about copper deficiency but to balance our zinc intake.

Our bodies need copper for the proper functioning of a number of important enzymes. One of these enzymes regulates pigment formation in the hair and skin. Farmers know that when the fleece of black sheep turns gray, it is often a sign of copper deficiency.

A more serious effect of copper deficiency can cause scarcity of neutrophils (a type of white blood cell) in humans, as well as neurologic disorders and vascular defects in young children. Such problems are rare, though, and occur only because of extreme malnutrition or malabsorption (as, for instance, in extensive stomach or colon resection or total unsupplemented intravenous nutrition).

On the other hand, excess copper is toxic, since free copper ions, not bound to other substances, react with oxygen and produce free radicals (just as iron ions do). In supplements, these metals are therefore combined with other molecules, as in copper salicylate, and are perfectly safe to take that way.

Chapter 20

Iron

The public has been oversold on the alleged need for iron supplements. Advertisers of iron-containing supplements especially target premenopausal women, instilling fear by exaggerating the possible consequences of marginal iron deficiencies. In reality, though, the small loss of iron during menstruation is quickly made up by the body itself.

At the same time, the risks of iron overload have been underplayed. Iron is, after all, a pro-oxidant. When it combines with oxygen-containing molecules in the body, it can generate destructive free radicals and cause the peroxidation of fats in cells and body tissue, or the destruction of red blood cells. It is therefore not a good idea to take iron supplements unless you know, on the strength of a laboratory test, that you are iron deficient.

As we explain in the chapter "Red Meat: Is It Worth the

Risk?" there are two types of iron––heme iron from meat (and other nonvegetarian supplements), which accumulates in the body and is dangerous in high concentrations, especially with regard to heart disease and strokes. On the other hand, the beneficial non-heme iron—from vegetarian sources, dairy products, and eggs—does not accumulate in the body.

Until now, people have been told that the "good" non-heme iron from nonmeat sources is poorly absorbed. The traditional reason given is that certain plant compounds—phytates, polyphenols, tannins, and oxalates—as well as calcium and phosphate bind to the non-heme iron and greatly reduce its absorption. Recently, however, large-scale studies with rural populations in China have shown this assumption to be wrong.

It was found that rural Chinese get negligible amounts of the readily absorbed heme iron, since they eat practically no red meat. On the other hand, they get plenty of the supposedly poorly absorbed non-heme iron from their basically vegetarian diet, several times as high in vegetables and grains as the traditional American/European diet.

So you would think that these people must be very low on iron—especially since they drink tea all day long, which is high in tannins that supposedly bind with non-heme iron and prevent its absorption. Yet, to everyone's surprise, all biochemical indicators of iron status (hemoglobin, plasma ferritin, and plasma iron-binding capacity) showed that these populations have perfectly normal iron levels.[1]

A further analysis concluded that "iron status is not compromised by a mainly vegetarian Chinese diet," and that there was "no suggestion that iron deficiency is a causal factor of anemia in this population."[2] Likewise, an analysis of data from several studies of Western vegetarian diets showed "no particular mineral deficiencies."[3]

Scientists admit that some biomarkers of mineral status in vegetarians, such as serum ferritin, are occasionally a bit low compared with nonvegetarian reference values.[4] But they also point out that these nonvegetarian iron levels "may, in fact, be undesirably high."[5] In short, there is nothing to indicate that if you reduce the risk of heart disease and cancer by drastically cutting back on meat and fat intake, you might thereby increase other health risks, such as creating mineral deficiencies. The smart and prudent thing to do, therefore, is to get our iron from nonmeat sources.*

NOTES

1. Chen, J., et al. Diet, life-style and mortality in China. A study of the characteristics of 65 Chinese counties. Ithaca, NY: Cornell University Press, 1990.
2. Beard, J. L., et al. Iron nurtriture in the Cornell-China diet cancer survey. *Am. J. Clin. Nutr.*, 1988; 47:771.
3. Kelsay, J. L., et al. Impact of variation in carbohydrate intake on mineral utilization by vegetarians. *Am. J. Clin. Nutr.*, 1988; 48:875–79.
   See also Frieland-Gravels, J., et al. Mineral adequacy of vegetarian diets. *Am. J. Clin. Nutr.*, 1988; 48: 859–62.
4. Dwyer, J. T., et al. Nutritional status of vegetarian children. *Am. J. Clin. Nutr.*, 1982; 35:204–16.
5. Campbell, T. C., et al. Diet and chronic degenerative diseases: perspectives from China. *Am. J. Clin. Nutr.*, 1994; 59S: 1153–61S.

*We recommend a vegetarian iron supplement—Floradix Iron + Herbs—from Flora. This product is carried by many health food stores. If unavailable, call 1-800-498-3610.

Chapter 21

POTASSIUM

Potassium's main role is in controlling blood pressure. In fact, we think the emphasis on low sodium intake to control essential hypertension—although fully justified—is much too one-sided. Even more important than excessive sodium intake (most of it from the overuse of table salt) is insufficient potassium intake. This is especially true for people on a meat-based diet, for meat provides much less potassium than vegetables. (Populations on vegetarian diets are known to have much less hypertension, heart disease, and stroke.)

What is most important is the potassium/sodium ratio, which should be in favor of potassium, but more often than not is in favor of sodium. In other words, it is not enough to reduce the consumption of table salt; it is equally important to supplement potassium to arrive at a better balance.

The potassium/sodium ratio is also an important factor in

cancer. An anticancer diet is high in vegetables and fruits, both of which are rich sources of potassium. However, even that is not enough when faced with special health risks like hypertension or cancer. For that reason, we take a small amount (100 mg/day) of supplemental potassium, although our diet is much richer in potassium than the average American/European diet.

Along with too little potassium intake, many people also do not get enough iodine from their diet. Even marginal iodine deficiencies can have far-reaching physical and emotional effects. The best food sources of iodine (as well as potassium) are saltwater fish, shellfish and, above all, sea vegetables (seaweeds), especially kelp fronds (kombu).

Part Four

Our Biological Supplements

Chapter 22

Flaxseed Oil

For a long time, we took only a tablespoon of flaxseed oil (but not borage oil), right after breakfast, together with our first Performance Pack of the day (see Chapter 3) and our hormonal supplements (DHEA for both of us and, in Phyllis's case, her three natural prescription estrogens (estradiol, estriol, and estrone) and progesterone. At the same time, we are taking our alpha lipoic acid (see Chapter 11) and coQ10 (see Chapter 12), which are, like the DHEA, best absorbed with some kind of lipid (fatty substance). Moreover, both alpha lipoic acid and coQ10 are ideal free radical quenchers for DHEA.

As to the type of flaxseed oil, we use only the kind that is high in "lignans,"* as that way you get the additional biofla-

*We get our "high lignan" flaxseed oil from Barlean's Organic Oils, Ferndale, Washington (1-800-445-FLAX) because of their very sophisticated

vonoids of the lignans from the shells of the flax seeds. Now, however, we also take ¼ teaspoon of borage oil, an addition we will explain shortly.

But let's first talk about flaxseed oil, which is undoubtedly the most important among medicinal plant oils.

Germany's famous "flaxseed lady," Dr. Johanna Budwig—M.D. and double Ph.D. in chemistry and physics, and two-time Nobel-prize nominee—suggests taking flaxseed oil, preferably with some yogurt or cottage cheese. She says these dairy foods contain certain milk proteins, which can combine with super-unsaturated oils, like flaxseed oil, borage oil, or primrose oil, to make them more water-soluble and hence more easily absorbable.

As Dr. Budwig explains, the way it works is like this: "When we analyze fats, we find fatty acid chains with eighteen segments. In some places, the chain is easily broken; it is loose and can absorb water. It is like roughing a smooth silk thread. The thread will absorb dye or water more easily where it has been roughed. It is specifically at these double bond sites that protein is readily incorporated. The fatty acid becomes water-soluble by combining with the protein."* So, whenever possible, we take an extra teaspoon or tablespoon of flaxseed oil with an after-dinner portion of low-fat yogurt.

Essential fatty acids, as in flaxseed oil, have several vital functions:

- to increase metabolic rate and improve metabolism
- to increase oxygen uptake

extraction process, which keeps peroxidation at a minimum. There are, however, other suppliers of flaxseed oil to choose from, which may be equally recommended. Recently we have also been buying flaxseeds from the same company (Barlean's), grinding them in a coffee mill, and adding a teaspoon of them to our cooked breakfast cereal.

*As cited in an interview with Tom Valentine in his *Health Letter,* Jan/Feb. 1993.

- to increase energy production (in the mitochondria of cells)
- to prevent cell membranes from "leaking," keeping harmful substances from getting into cells and beneficial ones from getting out
- they are required for the transport and metabolism of cholesterol and triglycerides
- they lower high cholesterol levels and triglycerides
- they are required for proper brain function (especially linolenic acid)
- they produce hormonelike substances called prostaglandins, which have important regulating functions in the body.*

Dr. Ralph Moss, in his book *Cancer Therapy,* notes that radiologists at the University of California at Los Angeles claim to have found surprisingly high concentrations of linoleic acid in the small intestines of mice. Since it has always been puzzling to researchers why cancer rarely develops in the small intestine, it is now believed that the presence of this fatty acid might be the protective factor. These researchers also found that the water-soluble form of linoleic acid (sodium linoleate) has a proclivity for killing leukemia cells.[1]

Other researchers at the University of Toronto point to the earlier mentioned lignans as the anticancer agents in flaxseed oil, particularly with respect to colon cancer. They said that their "test results suggest a protective effect of flaxseed on colon cancer risk at the promotional stage of carcinogenesis."[2]

As others have pointed out, flaxseed oil is a "concentrated source of plant lignans."[3] In the colon, these plant lignans are acted upon by bacteria and turned into mammalian lignans, which scientists credit with the anticancer effect of this oil.

*Prostaglandins, like the essential fatty acids from which they are made, serve important regulatory functions in the body, among them regulation of arterial muscle tone, sodium excretion via the urinary system, prevention of platelet stickiness in the blood, and regulating inflammatory response and immune functions.

Do not use flaxseed oil for cooking; the heat would instantly destroy all its therapeutic benefits. You can, however, use flaxseed oil for salad dressings, but in that case add some ascorbyl palmitate (the fat-soluble form of vitamin C) to prevent the air-exposed flaxseed oil from becoming oxidized.

Aside from all this, flaxseed oil—as well as ground flax seeds—have been shown to raise alpha-linolenic and long-chain n-3 (omega-3)* fatty acid levels in both blood plasma and erythrocytes (red blood cells) of humans. This resulted in lowering serum total cholesterol by 9% and low-density-lipoprotein cholesterol (LDL) by 18%. It also illustrates the high bioavailability of alpha-linolenic acid from either ground flaxseeds or flaxseed oil.[4]

NOTES

1. Norman, A., et al. Antitumor activity of sodium linoleate. *Nutr. Cancer*, 1988; 107–15.
2. Serraino, M., and L. U. Thompson. Flaxseed supplementation and early markers of colon carcinogenesis. *Cancer Letters*, 1992; 63:159–65.
3. Kurzer, M. S., et al. Fecal lignan and isoflavonoid excretion in premenopausal women consuming flaxseed powder. *Cancer Epidemiology, Biomarkers & Prevention*, June 1995; 4 (4): 353–58.
4. Cunnane, S. C., et al. High alpha-linolenic acid flaxseed (Linum usitatissimum): some nutritional properties in humans. *Br. J. Nutr.* (AZ4), Mar. 1993; 69(2): 443–53.

*N-3 or omega-3 fatty acids are also the dominant fats in fish oils, but flaxseed oil appears to be far superior, quite apart from being much better tasting.

Chapter 23

Borage Oil

The reason we take ¼ teaspoon of borage oil along with our flaxseed oil is that borage oil is the best source of gamma linolenic acid (GLA). Both flaxseed oil and borage oil are also good sources of linoleic acid, which the body normally converts into GLA. Some individuals, however, lack the enzyme that converts linoleic acid to GLA. Since testing whether we have or don't have this enzyme is difficult, it is good insurance to take some borage oil, for that reason alone.

Getting more GLA is also a good idea for many other reasons. For one thing, the body converts GLA into prostaglandin E1 (PGE1),[1] which regulates the production of a number of other prostaglandins. All of these have important functions, including control of arterial muscle tone[2] and sodium excretion through the kidneys. Most important, they prevent blood platelets from becoming "sticky" and forming dangerous blood clots in our arteries.

All of this adds up to GLA supplementation producing "significant reductions in blood pressure," as has been shown in a number of studies.[3] We therefore recommend borage oil, with its high content of GLA, to anyone suffering from high blood pressure—all the more so, since the usually prescribed, pharmaceutical drugs for high blood pressure can have nasty side effects, including impotence.

GLA is also of great importance for diabetics. According to a recent study, supplementation with GLA was able to reduce the severity of the discomfiting neuropathies—painful sensations or numbness in hands and feet—that often accompany advanced diabetes.[4] Since diabetics are frequently also overweight and suffer from high blood pressure, there is all the more reason why diabetics should include borage oil in their nutritional supplement program.

Last but not least, GLA, when provided as a dietary supplement, has been reported to improve clinical symptoms of several inflammatory disorders. A recent study has confirmed this effect,[5] which should be of great interest to all those suffering from such chronic inflammatory conditions as arthritis, rheumatoid arthritis, Crohn's disease, and similar inflammatory bowel conditions.*

NOTES

1. Fan, Y. Y., and R. S. Chapkin. Mouse peritoneal macrophage prostaglandin E1 synthesis is altered by dietary gamma-linolenic acid. *Journal of Nutrition,* Aug. 1992; 122 (8): 1600–1606.
2. Fan, Y. Y., R. S. Chapkin, and K. S. Ramos. Dietary lipid source alters murine macrophage/vascular smooth muscle cell interactions in vitro. *Journal of Nutrition,* Sept. 1996; 126 (9): 2083–88.
3. Engler, M. M. Comparative study of diets enriched with evening primrose, black currant, borage and fungal oils on blood pressure and pressor

*GLA (gamma linolenic acid) is also available as a supplement (240 mg caps containing 24% GLA; Vitamin Research Products 1-800-877-2447).

responses in spontaneously hypertensive rats. *Prostaglandins, Leukotrienes & Essential Fatty Acids,* Oct. 1993; 49 (4): 809–14.

4. Keen, H., and J. Payen. Treatment of diabetic neuropathy with gamma linolenic acid. *Diabetes Care,* 1993; 16 (1): 8–15.
5. Chilton-Lopez, S., D. D. Swan, A. N. Fonteh, M. M. Johnson, and F. H. Chilton. Metabolism of gammalinolenic acid in human neutrophils. *Journal of Immunology,* Apr. 15, 1996; 156 (8): 2941–47.

Chapter 24

Bioflavonoids, Phenols, and Carotenoids

We get the extra bioflavonoids we don't get from our diet either in lignan-containing flaxseed oil or by taking two capsules of proanthocyanidins,* another powerful type of bioflavonoids.

In vitro proanthocyanidins are said to have fifty times greater antioxidant capability than vitamin C. We do not know whether that is so in the live system, as well, but they definitely help, working in tandem with glutathione, to restore oxidized vitamin C to its fresh antioxidant state.

Still another way of getting bioflavonoids would be to take Bioflavonoid Complex tablets, or some liquid flavonoid extract. The plant kingdom produces many different kinds of biofla-

*Proanthocyanidins are, for instance, available from the Life Extension Foundation (1-800-544-4440).

vonoids, some of the best-known ones being quercetin and rutin, as well as the hesperidin complex.*

These plant chemicals are present in the mostly nonedible parts of fruits, such as the white pulp of oranges and lemons. They are, however, also present in other biological sources, such as blue-green algae and, in the form of catechin, in green tea, which we thoroughly enjoy on a daily basis.

Likewise, the antioxidant pycnogenol, extracted from either grape pits or the bark of the marine pine tree, which many people are taking because of its antioxidant properties, is technically a bioflavonoid.

Why do we take bioflavonoids? For one thing, bioflavonoids are known for their cell membrane–stabilizing effect. Half a century ago, the famous Hungarian scientist and Nobel laureate Dr. Szent-Györgyi was the first to notice this effect in the course of work that led to the discovery of vitamin C. A friend of his had asked if he knew of anything that might help with his bleeding gums. Dr. Szent-Györgyi let him have some of the plant extract from which he was trying to isolate ascorbic acid (vitamin C), thinking that the vitamin might heal the man's gums.

The man's gums were healed all right, but not by the vitamin C. That became clear later when Dr. Szent-Györgyi gave the man some purified vitamin C, and it did no good. Rather, it turned out that the healing effect resulted from the "contaminants" in the raw, unpurified vitamin C. And what were these "contaminants"? You guessed it—the compounds that became known as "bioflavonoids."

Cell membrane stability and integrity is, of course, very important for the smooth and controlled exchange of nutrients, gases, and fluids between the exterior and interior of cells. If cell membranes become "leaky" and this delicate mechanism stops

*Any good health food store should have at least two or three brands of bioflavonoid products to choose from. Vitamin Research Products (1-800-877-2447) also offers a well-balanced bioflavonoid complex, containing rutin, quercetin, and hesperidin complex.

functioning properly, all kinds of things can go wrong. For instance, invading bacteria and viruses can get into cells whose membranes are no longer intact and therefore cannot provide a protective shield against such parasites.

Bioflavonoids also seem to have antiviral effect. This is of special importance in viral-related cancers, such as certain leukemias and papillary carcinomas (for instance, of the cervix). Any harmless, natural substance like bioflavonoids, which holds out reasonable promise (even if no definite proof) of having an antiviral effect, should therefore be welcome in such cases.

Also, bioflavonoids have been found to be effective *in vitro* against the herpes type 1 virus and a number of the so-called rhinoviruses that cause the common cold. It would therefore be a good idea—assuming that this *in vitro* effect also occurs *in vivo,* that is, in the live organism—not only to increase vitamin C intake to fight a cold but to simultaneously take bioflavonoids.

In test tube studies, quercetin and other bioflavonoids have also been shown to be anti-inflammatory, although this effect has, as of this writing, not yet been demonstrated by *in vivo* studies in animals and humans.

Chapter 25

Modified Citrus Pectin

One can call modified citrus pectin another type of bioflavonoid, since it is made from the soluble component of citrus fruit fiber.

We are not taking this supplement right now, because there seems to be no need for it. But for anyone who has cancer with a risk of metastasis, this supplement should be seriously considered, though it is rather pricey.

But, then, anything that might prevent metastasis is "priceless" anyway—provided one can afford it.

Modified citrus pectin's antimetastatic effects are fairly well documented. Earlier studies had already shown antimetastatic effects of modified citrus pectin for different types of cancer in both animal and human studies, for instance, in the case of colorectal cancer and melanoma.[1] A recent animal study with orally administered modified citrus pectin has shown it to be "a potent inhibitor of spontaneous prostate carcinoma metastasis."[2]

The important point, however, is that, independent of the type and site of the primary tumor, modified citrus pectin seems to be able to inhibit the adhesion of metastatic cancer cells to the epithelial cells of target organs.

The way this works is complicated, but briefly put, cancer cells produce an excess of galactose-binding lectins, which become proteins on the malignant cell surface. These lectin proteins are necessary for the metastatic cancer cells to attach themselves to the blood vessel walls of any organ with which they come into contact, in order to form secondary tumors. The pectin fragments of modified citrus pectin, however, deprive cancer cells of using this "trick" and thereby can prevent the formation of secondary tumors.

Shark cartilage is known to have a similar antimetastatic effect, but for quite a different reason. Research shows that shark cartilage can, to a certain extent, deprive tumors of their blood supply, thus making them shrink and eventually die. In the same way, shark cartilage can apparently prevent new tumors from metastasizing. At least, this is potentially possible. The 15% average success rate for shark cartilage with various cancers is, however, not impressive. Also, rather large amounts of it have to be taken to produce any effect. It seems, thus, that—if the idea is to prevent metastasis—modified citrus pectin is a more promising natural substance for that purpose.*

*Recent studies have shown combination therapy with the two antiangiostatic (i.e., new-blood-vessel-inhibiting) drugs—*endostatin* and *angiostatin*—to be effective in the suppression of metastasis. (See also Dr. Robert Nagourney's remarks about them, pages 297–299.)

NOTES

1. Irimura, T., Y. Matsushita, R. C. Sutton, et al. Increased content of an endogenous lactose-binding lectin in human colorectal carcinoma progressed to metastatic stages. *Cancer Res.*, 1991; 51: 387–393.

   Platt, D., and A. Raz. Modulation of the lung colonization of B16-F1 melanoma cells by citrus pectin. *J. Natl. Cancer Inst.*, 1992; 84-438442.
2. Pienta, K. J., H. Naic, A. Akhtar, et al. Inhibition of spontaneous metastasis in a rat prostate cancer model by oral administration of modified citrus pectin. *J. Natl. Cancer Inst.*, 1995; 87: 348–353.

Chapter 26

Curcumin (Essence of Turmeric)

Curcumin, the beautiful, sun-yellow active ingredient of the spice turmeric (*Curcuma longa*), is perhaps the most important health-protective plant chemical of all. In fact, the powdered rhizome or root of the turmeric plant itself, from which curcumin is derived, has been used in the ancient Ayurvedic system of Indian medicine for thousands of years for a variety of illnesses such as stomach problems, indigestion, flatulence (gas), urinary tract infections, and skin diseases.

Curcumin's chemical structure, a natural phenolic compound, was already discovered in 1910, but it was not until the mid-1970s and 1980s that scientists came to appreciate its many other antioxidant and anti-inflammatory uses. Today, the spice turmeric and its active ingredient, curcumin, are—because of their unique antioxidant and anti-inflammatory properties—among the best researched herbal medicines worldwide.

Curcumin's Antioxidant Properties

Curcumin—a collective term for the three "curcuminoids" it encompasses—has been shown to be a very effective inhibitor of such tissue-destroying oxygen fragments as superoxide and hydroxyl radicals.[1] However, as Muhammed Majeed, Ph.D., and Vladimir Badmaev, M.D., have pointed out, curcumin—unlike other antioxidants that have a more direct, "policing effect" on free radicals and scavenge and neutralize them in head-on confrontation—the turmeric curcuminoids go "under cover." They merge with the free-radical troublemakers, rather than fight them, and thereby absorb and neutralize many of their destructive characteristics, even before they have a chance to become active.[2]

Curcumin is hence especially effective in preventing peroxidation of lipids, that is, preventing fats and oils from becoming rancid. Moreover, they do so in a benign, natural, and nontoxic way—a purpose for which the food industry is still, by and large, depending on the synthetic phenolics BHT and BHA, which are potentially toxic.

Since the oxidation of fats and oils is facilitated by the presence of iron ions, it is interesting to note that curcumin, just like the earlier discussed flavonoids—catechin, quercetin, and others—is able to chelate (bind) iron and thus remove it via urinary excretion from the body—another way of preventing the formation of lipid peroxides.[3]

Curcumin's Anti-Inflammatory Properties

It is impossible to separate curcumin's antioxidant properties from its anti-inflammatory ones, because inflammation is, in large part, due to the chemical warfare waged by immune system cells, using nitric oxide and other oxygen compounds against invading organisms, such as bacteria and viruses.

Usually, steroidal drugs like cortisone or nonsteroidal anti-inflammatory drugs, like phenylbutazone and indomethacin, are used to treat inflammations. The trouble is that both of these types of drugs have undesirable side effects, including a weakening of the immune system.

In contrast, curcumin has been shown in animal and human studies to have the same anti-inflammatory effects as these harsher, immunity-suppressing drugs—and without all the bad side effects.

In one study, for instance, one group of surgery patients received standard, postoperative treatment with the steroidal drug phenylbutazone to combat inflammation and to aid in wound healing, while another group received only curcumin. The result: curcumin was just as effective in reducing postoperative inflammation as the much less desirable drug phenylbutazone.[4]

Oral curcumin has also proved effective in a rat experiment, in controlling artificially induced osteoarthritis and the inflammation that is typically part of it.[5]

Curcumin, at an oral dose of 1,200 mg/day, was also tested in a double-blind trial in forty-nine patients with rheumatoid arthritis. Within five to six weeks, there was "significant improvement" in all patients, including reduced morning stiffness and improvement in physical endurance, similar to the group receiving phenylbutazone.[6]

It is also now understood by what mechanism curcumin and its three "curcuminoids" produce these anti-inflammatory effects. Put briefly and in the simplest possible terms, curcumin inhibits a cascade of inflammatory events from the metabolic breakdown of an unsaturated fatty acid called arachidonic acid. This cascade of biochemical events produces such inflammatory products as prostaglandins, leukotrienes and similar compounds, all of which have inflammatory effects.

By interfering with this process, curcumin acts pretty much like aspirin and other anti-inflammatory drugs. What gives curcumin the edge over these types of drugs, though, is that—contrary to them—it does not simultaneously affect the synthesis of prostacyclin, which we need to prevent platelet build-up in our arteries and to keep them well dilated so blood can circulate freely throughout the body. That makes curcumin the anti-inflammatory therapy of choice for those at risk of vascular thrombosis.

Curcumin's Anticancer Properties

Turmeric, in spice form, and curcumin have been shown to be anticarcinogenic in a number of animal experiments and a few human trials. Turmeric has been shown to inhibit benzopyrene-induced stomach and mammary tumors in mice.[7] Likewise, curcumin in the diet of rats inhibited the process leading to the development of colon cancer.[8]

In one clinical study involving one hundred patients with oral cancer, 500 mg of curcumin taken three times a day for thirty days greatly improved their condition.[9] In another clinical study, 1,500 mg of curcumin a day was administered (in divided doses) for thirty days to sixteen chronic smokers in India.

As a result, there was considerably less urinary excretion of tobacco-related mutagens in these people, showing that curcumin therapy is able to counteract smoking-induced mutagenesis and carcinogenesis.[10] An aqueous extract of the spice turmeric also inhibited the action of smoking-related mutagens.[11]

In light of the above-mentioned studies, smokers who are not yet able to stop smoking are well advised to take curcumin supplements (along with other antimutagenic and anticarcinogenic supplements).

Another experiment revealed a unique mode of action of cucurmin—similar to the tumor-suppressing drugs *endostatin* and *angiostatin*—whereby it effectively prevented the formation of new blood vessels in proliferating cells, without which there can be no tumor formation. The scientists therefore concluded that "[curcumin] could turn out to be a very useful compound for the development of novel anticancer therapy."[12] At a minimum, curcumin should, in our opinion, be used to support chemotherapy and radiation therapy.

Curcumin and AIDS

Curcumin is currently undergoing intensive study as a "biological response modifier," that is, as a natural means of bolstering the immune system.

A preliminary clinical report on the results of curcumin therapy for HIV-infected patients was presented in 1994 at the International Conference on AIDS in San Francisco. In that pilot study, eighteen HIV-positive volunteers were given 2,000 mg of oral curcumin per day for approximately twenty weeks. Of this group, eleven patients had clinical symptoms of HIV infection, while seven persons were symptom free.

In this case, curcumin therapy alone, without any other medication, resulted in a significant increase in CD-4 and CD-8 cell counts, as compared to the matched control group, which had received a dummy pill. The scientists involved in this study therefore concluded that curcumin is a safe and effective treatment to raise lymphocyte counts in HIV-infected patients.[13]

In another, slightly later study, curcumin was able to inhibit the activity of the enzyme integrase, which HIV requires to penetrate into CD-4 and CD-8 lymphocytes.[14] This, then, seems to be the mechanism by which curcumin helps to prevent the destruction of these immune system cells.

Still another laboratory study from Rutgers University suggests that curcumin is able to inhibit the production of inflammatory cytokines like tumor necrosis factor and interleukin-1, among others, all of which promote HIV build-up in cells.[15] (Incidentally, this mechanism may, at least in part, explain curcumin's general, anti-inflammatory effect.)

Other Protective Effects of Curcumin

Curcuminoids in extracts from turmeric were found to inhibit the growth of many gram positive and gram negative bacteria, fungi, and even the intestinal parasite, *Entamoeba histolytica,* which causes amoebic dysentery.[16]

Curcumin is also able to reverse liver damage caused by mold poisons (aflatoxins).[17]

Furthermore, an animal study found cucumin as effective in preventing lack of blood flow to the heart muscle after heart attack as the standard heart drug quinidine.[18]

Still another unexpected effect of curcumin concerns its protective function with regard to cataract formation (at least it did so in a mixed *in vivo* and *in vitro* study with rat lenses).[19]

The researchers concluded that this protective effect was due to the observed fact of curcumin increasing the antioxidant enzyme system glutathione-S-transferase in the rat lenses. Since cataract formation is the result of free radical activity in the lens, and since this enzyme system is also one of our own main antioxidant defense systems, curcumin should also have a protective effect with regard to cataract formation in the human lens.

NOTES

1. Reddy, A. C. P., and B. R. Lokesh. Studies on spice principles as antioxidants in the inhibition of lipid peroxidation of rat liver microsomes. *Mol. Cell. Biochem.,* 1992; 111–117.
2. Majeed, M., and V. Badmaev. *Turmeric and the healing curcuminoids.* New Canaan, Conn: Keats Publishing, 1996.
3. Sreejayan, and M. N. Rao. Curcuminoids as potent inhibitors of lipid peroxidation. *J. Pharmacy & Pharmacology,* Dec. 1994; 46 (12): 1013–16.
4. Satoskar, R. R., et al. Evaluation of anti-inflammatory property of curcumin in patients with post-operative inflammation. *Ind. J. Clin. Pharmacol. Toxicol.,* 1986; 24:651.
5. Srimal, R. C., and B. N. Dhawan. Pharmacological and clinical studies on curcuma longa. *Hamdard Natl. Found. Monograph,* New Delhi, India, Section 3B (ii); 131.
6. Deodhar, S. D., et al. Preliminary studies on anti-rheumatic activity of curcumin. *Ind. J. Med. Res.,* 1980; 71: 632.
7. Nagabhushan, M., and S. V. Bhide. Antimutagenicity and anticarcinogenicity of turmeric. *J. Nutr. Growth Canc.,* 1987; 4:83.

   Nagabhushan, M. Ph.D. diss., University of Bombay, India, 1987.
8. Rao, C. V., et al. Inhibition by dietary curcumin of azoxymethane-induced ornithine decarboxylase, tyrosine protein kinase, arachidonic

acid metabolism and aberrant crypt foci formation in the rat colon. *Carcinogenesis,* 1993; 14: 2219.

Rao, C. V., et al. Chemoprevention of colon carcinogenesis by dietary curcumin, a naturally occurring plant phenolic compound. *Cancer Res.,* 1995; 55: 259.

9. Turmeric's anti-cancer use. Press release (UNI), Hyderabad, India, 1992.
10. Polasa, K., et al. Effect of turmeric on urinary mutagens in smokers. *Mutagenesis,* 1992; 7: 107.
11. Azuine, M. A., et al. Protective role of aqueous turmeric extract against mutagenicity of firet-acting carcinogens as well as benzo (alpha) pyrene-induced genotoxicity and carcinogenicity." *J. Canc. Res. Clin. Oncol.,* 1992; 118: 447.
12. Singh, A. K., et al. Curcumin inhibits the proliferation and cell cycle progression of human umbilical vein endothelial cell. *Cancer Letters,* Oct. 1, 1996; 107(1): 109–15.
13. Copeland, R., D. Baker, and I. Wilson. Curcumin therapy in HIV-infected patients initially increased CD-4 and CD-8 cell counts (abstract No. PB0876) *Intern. Conf. AIDS,* 1994; 10(2): 216.
14. Mazunder, A., et al. Inhibition of human immunodeficiency virus type-1 integrase by curcumin. *Biochem. Pharmacol.,* 1995; 49(8): 1165–70.
15. Chan, M-Y., et al. Inhibition of tumor necrosis by curcumin, a phytochemical. *Biochem. Pharmacol.,* 49(11): 1551–56.
16. Ammon, H. P. T., and M. A. Wahl. Pharmacology of curcuma longa. *Planta Med.,* 1991; 57:1.
17. Soni, K. B., et al. Reversal of aflatoxin-induced liver damage by turmeric and curcumin. *Cancer Lett.,* 1992; 66: 115.
18. Dikshit, M., et al. Prevention of ischaemia-induced biochemical changes in curcumin and quinidine in the cat heart. *Ind. J. Med. Res.,* 1995; 101: 31–35.
19. Awasthi, S., et al. Curcumin protects against 4-hydroxy-2-trans-nonenal-induced cataract formation in rat lenses. *Am. J. Clin. Nutr.,* Nov. 1996; 64(S): 761–66.

Chapter 27

Yohimbine: Nature's Answer to Viagra

When all the hullabaloo about the impotency pill Viagra exploded in the American media, and men by the thousands clamored for prescriptions for the $10-a-shot pill, it gave us a weird feeling of unreality. Viagra, the first medicine for impotency? Hadn't anybody noticed that there had all along been a perfectly natural impotency remedy called yohimbine? (We even called attention to it in the first edition of *Formula for Life*.) Yet, yohimbine has remained one of nature's best kept secrets.

Yohimbine really works as well as or perhaps even better than Viagra, and it is much cheaper and doesn't require a prescription.

It strikes us therefore as strange to see Viagra and similar drugs touted by multimillion-dollar advertising and P.R., as if they were the first and only cures for impotency—that is, "erectile dysfunction," to be politically correct. Tell that to native African healers ("witch doctors") or South American shamans, who have been treating this distressing affliction of men for centuries with concoctions from the bark of the West African *yohimbe* tree (*Corynanthe yohimbe*) or its South American equivalent, popularly known as *quebracho blanco (Aspidosperma quebracho).*

Yohimbine, as a natural impotency treatment, would not have been news to men in Victorian England either, where it was brought from the African colonies and referred to, tongue-in-cheek, as "the refuge of aging Don Juans."

In this country, though, American health food stores did not start selling capsules with dried extract of yohimbine or little bottles with yohimbine extract until just a few years ago. Also, yohimbine is less widely known here because supplement manufacturers—unlike drug companies—are not allowed to make "health claims" for natural products. So how would people know what yohimbine was good for? It didn't help matters that some unscrupulous manufacturers "forgot" to put genuine yohimbine into their "yohimbine" products. No wonder the deceived customers who had been taking nothing more than sugar pills concluded that yohimbine doesn't work.

Some products, though, do contain honest-to-goodness yohimbine and *do* work. One of them is YohimbeMax (a capsule containing 1,000 mg of dried yohimbe bark extract, with some Damiana and a little ginseng, dong quai, vitamin E, and zinc picolinate thrown in for good measure, which may sound impressive, but probably adds nothing important to the main ingredient). We know of several men who have consistently had good results with this product. (Two to three 1,000 mg capsules, one hour before sexual relations, seems to be a reasonable average dose.)*

The product we have used for several years, though—not only for its sex-enhancing effects but also for its mental benefits—

*YohimbeMax also exists as a 1,500 mg capsule. We are told, however, that this extra-large capsule is difficult to swallow.

is a liquid extract of African yohimbe bark.* We like the liquid form best, mainly because it acts faster (approximately thirty minutes, compared with forty-five to sixty minutes for the capsules). Besides, it is easier to fine-tune the right individual amount trying with a few drops more, or a few drops less, at a time. (For most people, twenty to thirty drops one hour before sexual relations should be a good starting dose.)

As with most chemical compounds, whether natural or pharmaceutical, body weight is also a factor: a 170-pound man may need more than, say, a 145-pound one or a 120-pound woman (yes, it works for women, too, but more about that later). Also, we metabolize chemicals differently; so the right dose for one person may be too much or too little for another.

Also, experience has shown that yohimbine is absorbed twice as fast when taken on an empty stomach instead of after a heavy meal (common sense suggests that making love on a full stomach is obviously not a good idea anyway).

Nor is it advisable ever to take more than 50% above the normal dose as indicated on the label. If that still does not do the trick, yohimbine just may not be nature's solution for you. (In that case, there is always Viagra and nothing much has been lost.)

On the other hand, if yohimbine works for you—and it works for most men who have only intermittent potency problems and even for about 25% of those with serious chronic potency disturbances (like, for instance, diabetic impotency)—consider yourself lucky. Also, several men of our own acquaintance, who are anything but impotent, still use yohimbine. They do so, they say, because it enlarges the penis beyond normal size and maintains the erection for longer periods of time, as has also been our own experience.

Although Viagra may do the same, natural, nonprescription yohimbine is so much cheaper and, besides, has certain func-

*There is more than one supplier of yohimbe extract; we are using a double macerated one from Gaia Herbs (1-800-831-7780). A 4-ounce trial bottle would be a sensible starting order.

tional advantages. There is, first of all, yohimbine's mood-elevating and energizing effects. There is nothing better than a little yohimbine to pull one out of a midafternoon or early-evening slump. We may use it, for instance, when putting in long hours of library research or writing. It seems to make for greater clarity of thought and helping one to get more done. But frankly, we also notice that, by speeding things up, one tends to make a few more mechanical mistakes, like striking the wrong key on the computer. Still, we think yohimbine's mental benefits far outweigh this minor downside.

Furthermore, yohimbine does not have some of Viagra's disadvantages. For instance, with yohimbine, your partner's skin will definitely not suddenly take on a "bluish hue," as happens with three in one-hundred Viagra cases (a real turn-off, if you ask us!). More important, with yohimbine there does not seem to be much danger from interactions with other drugs, about which one hears so much with regard to Viagra.

For instance, it strikes us as a bit weird that anyone obliged to carry nitroglycerine around because of imminent danger of heart attack would want to risk his life for a few minutes of sexual pleasure. Some people say, "What a great way to go!" But we find that logic hard to follow.

Which brings us to a more important point about side effects: yohimbine, too, tends to raise blood pressure, which definitely rules it out for *anyone* with hypertension. Also, those with kidney or liver disease should not take it.

Nor should severely disturbed mental patients (psychotics) take yohimbine. It can affect the central nervous system, which is also why—unlike Viagra—it has the above-mentioned mental energizing and mood-elevating effects, but it seems to adversely affect the brains of psychotics.

On the other hand, our clients who suffer from moderate and even severe depression or bipolar mood disturbances, and who use yohimbine for potency-enhancement, seem to have no negative side effects. Yohimbine is a natural antidepressant, but the heightened potency and more satisfactory sexual experiences are also bound to have mood-elevating effects.

In this connection, we hear that many men do not tell their female partners that they are taking either yohimbine or Viagra. The rationale is that the woman wants to feel that it is she who is responsible for the man's passion, not some chemical compound. In some cases (vanity being what it is) that may be so. One suspects, though, that the male ego does not want to admit to any outside help either.

How Do Viagra and Yohimbine Work?

Viagra and yohimbine work very differently. When a healthy, sexually functioning man is aroused, his brain sends signals to nerve cells all around the penis. These nerve cells then release nitric oxide, which in turn causes the penis to make another compound, called cyclic GMP (cGMP). Its function is to dilate blood vessels in the penis, allowing blood to rush in, resulting in the engorgement that is necessary for an erection.

Now, as long as the man remains in a state of arousal, he keeps producing this sexy compound cGMP, and as long as he is producing it, he will have an erection. The trouble is, at the same time, the body also produces an enzyme called phosphodiesterase 5 (PDE5) that destroys the erection-producing cGMP. But as long as there is enough sexual stimulation, the two natural compound keeps each other more or less in equilibrium, and the man maintains his erection.

However, if stimulation flags, the erection-destroying PDE5 gets the upper hand, and the man will lose his erection. That's exactly where Viagra comes into play: it prevents the "bad" PDE5 from destroying the "good" cGMP, thus giving the penis a chance to remain erect. Eventually, though, as with all good things, this benign mechanism comes to an end. And a jolly good thing, too, for without this safety mechanism a man would wind up with an erection lasting many hours—a most unpleasant and often painful condition called priapism.

Yohimbine, on the other hand, works very differently. It also brings blood down into the pelvic region, but it does so by blocking certain nerve receptors on the vascular smooth muscle in the whole genital area, thus causing blood vessels to dilate and expand. It also causes the myriad little valves that control blood flow in the spongy tissue of the penis to open properly and let the blood enter and then shuts them so the blood does not flow out prematurely, which would make the man lose his erection.

Unlike Viagra, however, yohimbine also has a direct central nervous system effect. It increases circulating levels of certain brain chemicals—catecholamines, including norepinephrine—known as "the brain's adrenaline." These "neurotransmitters" affect, first of all, the sympathetic nervous system, causing the expansion of blood vessels necessary for an erection. But they also cause other physiological effects, like a rise in blood pressure (a risk factor for people with hypertension) and increased respiration rate. That's the bad news; the good news is that these same brain chemicals also positively influence mood and desire, apparently including sexual desire.*

In these mental and emotional effects of yohimbine lies perhaps its biggest difference from Viagra. All the medical literature about the new "wonder drug" stresses the fact that Viagra does not affect a man's libido. In other words, if the man is not stimulated by outside influences—a sexy partner, erotic fantasies, or sexual imagery—Viagra does not work. Its manufacturer, Pfizer, keeps emphasizing over and over again that the little blue diamond-shaped pill is not an aphrodisiac—it does *not* stimulate desire!

Yohimbine, as we have seen, also brings blood into the pelvic area, as does Viagra, albeit by a different mechanism. In addition, however, yohimbine controls the many little valves (arterial sphincters) that regulate blood flow within the penis, something Viagra apparently does not do. Furthermore, in contrast to Viagra, yohimbine also influences mood and desire, be-

*Grasing, K., et al. Effects of yohimbine on autonomic measures are determined by individual values for area under the concentration-time curve. *J. Clin. Pharmacol.*, 1996; 36: 814–22.

cause of its central nervous system effect. It is this property of yohimbine that makes it—in total contrast to Viagra—a genuine aphrodisiac.

Do Yohimbine and Viagra Also Work for Women?

The $64,000 question is whether yohimbine and Viagra also work for women. In the case of Viagra, it would mean that—in the presence of sexual stimulation—the woman's clitoris (like the man's penis) does get engorged as long as cGMP dilates its blood vessels. That may well be so; but it still would not be a "turn on" for the woman. For that to happen, there must first be vaginal lubrication, the first sign of sexual arousal.

The onset of sexual arousal is exactly what many women who have taken yohimbine have experienced. It is also what co-author Phyllis Kronhausen has experienced herself many times (occasionally to her own distraction, when having taken a small amount of yohimbine for nonsexual purposes, such as keeping her mind alert while working). In a word, while the jury is still out, at this writing, on whether Viagra can do anything for women (it probably does), the experiential evidence is already in about yohimbine: it definitely can have a sexually stimulating effect for women, although not quite as dramatic as for men.

On the other hand, yohimbine—because of its effect on pelvic engorgement—helps a woman build what sex researchers Masters and Johnson call an "orgasmic platform." It seems therefore that, with yohimbine, Mother Nature has not been totally partial to men, but has thought of women, too.

Part Five

Our Supplemental Hormone Program

Chapter 28

MELATONIN

We are both taking 6 mg (two capsules of 3 mg each) of melatonin at bedtime. This is a reasonable, preventive dose, as well as a sleeping aid, but also has other, health-protective effects, as we will discuss.

Melatonin is a hormone produced by the pineal body, a small gland in the front and center of the brain. (This may be the origin of the "third eye" in Hindu mythology, marked by the traditional red dot that devout Hindus paint on their foreheads.)

The pineal gland and its hormone, melatonin—although of great importance to the physiology of both sexes—are of even greater importance to the well-being of women than of men. Their main function during the pubertal development of girls is to regulate the maturation of the female sexual organs. During the reproductive phase, melatonin seems to act as a "coordi-

WARNING: Melatonin should NOT be used by people with leukemia, Hodgkin's disease, lymphoma, or multiple myeloma. Paradoxically and by complicated, not fully understood mechanisms, melatonin could worsen these conditions.

nating signal" for the menstrual cycle. Finally, later in a woman's life, the pineal gland's declining output of melatonin determines the onset and course of the menopause, a decline which has been implicated as a factor in causing breast cancer.

In adult life, melatonin influences the wake/sleep pattern of both sexes, because the pineal gland secretes melatonin according to light conditions, transmitted to the brain via our visual system. From there, this information is passed on to almost every part of our physiology, such as the endocrine (hormonal) system, central nervous system, and immune system, thereby enabling body functions to adjust to the time of day and season.

In the mid-1980s, researchers Alfred Lewy and Robert L. Sack began to investigate whether it is possible to simulate the effects of darkness, that is, to set the body clock forward or backward, by giving people oral doses of melatonin. They discovered that melatonin pills could "trick" the body into "thinking" that dusk comes sooner, so people become sleepy earlier. "It's a natural sleeping pill that shifts the body clock in the desired direction," said Dr. Lewy, a professor of psychiatry, ophthalmology, and pharmacology at Oregon Health Sciences University.[1]

Researchers of the Massachusetts Institute of Technology confirmed these findings. They reported that their subjects dropped into deep sleep much faster after being given melatonin pills at bedtime: "Our volunteers fall asleep in five or six minutes on melatonin, while those on placebo take about fifteen minutes or longer."[2]

There now exists a new formulation of melatonin, specifically designed to enhance its sleep-promoting effects. The product contains several other micronutrients, the most important of which is pyridoxal 5-phosphate (a nonstimulating vitamin B-6 analog), which converts the amino acid tryptophan from foods into serotonin, a sleep-inducing hormone. If one, then, drinks a glass of warm milk or eats a slice of turkey breast about an hour before bedtime, the tryptophan from the milk or turkey meat is converted into sleep-inducing serotonin, thereby augmenting the effects of melatonin.*

Frankly, the sleep-inducing and sleep-improving effect of low-dose melatonin alone (6 mg in our case) is perfectly sufficient reason for our using it on a regular basis.† There is, however, also a proven anticancer effect of melatonin, which is another good reason for anyone at special cancer risk to take it.

As with many protective substances that our bodies produce, melatonin production declines with age, while the risk of cancer goes up. Consequently, anyone with a cancer history, or at special cancer risk, would be well advised to bed down with the help of some melatonin.

Melatonin has proven itself especially effective against estrogen-dependent breast cancer.[3] But its anticancer effect seems to be much more general; as one group of researchers put it, "Melatonin might prove to be a natural oncostatic [cancer-inhibiting] agent of practical value in cancer prevention."[4]

Following is a summary of international research findings about melatonin with respect to cancer protection:

- "Serum melatonin is depressed in patients with primary mammary cancer and experimental tumors are inhibited, a finding suggesting a therapeutic potential of melatonin."[5]

*The melatonin product referred to here is sold by the Life Extension Foundation (1-800-544-4440) under the trade name Natural Sleep. It also contains several other supporting nutrients, including niacinamide (vitamin B-3) and inositol, which also tend to reinforce melatonin's relaxing effects.

†Our sources for 3 mg melatonin capsules are either the Life Extension Foundation (1-800-544-4440) or Vitamin Research Products (1-800-877-2447).

- Serum melatonin levels are "significantly higher in (breast cancer) patients with the best prognosis for estrogen receptor–positive/node-negative cases."[6]
- Melatonin augments the effectiveness of Tamoxifen, a drug routinely given to estrogen-dependent breast cancer patients.[7]

Melatonin is definitely immunity-enhancing. As a group of Italian researchers put it, "one of the main targets of melatonin is the thymus, i.e., the central organ of the immune system."[8] These scientists therefore concluded that "in general, melatonin seems to have an immuno-enhancing effect that is particularly apparent in immunodepressive states [as, for instance, with cancer, HIV infection, and advanced age]."

This immuno-enhancing effect of melatonin was especially pronounced when combined with interleuken-2 therapy. One group of researchers found, for instance, that the "mean number of lymphocytes and eosinophils significantly increased during [melatonin/interleuken-2] treatment."[9]

A similar study found that "a single daily injection of low-dose IL-2 [interleuken-2] is able to efficiently activate lymphocyte proliferation in cancer patients when it is given in association with the pineal hormone MLT [melatonin]."[10] In that study, there was a significant increase in mean number of lymphocytes, T-lymphocytes, NK (natural killer) cells, CD25-positive cells and eosinophils—in short, an across-the-board boost in cellular imunity.

NOTES

1. As reported in *Harvard Health Letter,* a publication of Harvard Medical School, vol. 18, no. 8, June 1993.
2. As reported in *USA Today,* 1 March 1994.
3. Hill, S. M., L. L. Spriggs, M. A. Simon, et al. The growth-inhibitory action of melatonin on human breast cancer cells is linked to the estrogen response system. *Cancer Lett.,* July 10, 1992; 64 (3): 249–56.
4. Coleman, M. P., and R. J. Reiter. Breast cancer, blindness and melatonin. *Europ. J. Cancer,* 1992; 28 (203):501–503.

5. Bartsch, C., H. Bartsch, and T. H. Lippert. Role of the pineal body in reproduction and in gynecologic tumors. *Geburtshilfe & Frauenheilkunde* Jan. 1991; 51 (1): 1–8.
6. Barni, S., P. Lissoni, A. Ssormani, F. Pelizzoni, F. Brivio, S. Crispino, and G. Tancini. The pineal gland and breast cancer: serum levels of melatonin in patients with mammary tumors and their relation to clinical characteristics. *Int. J. Biol. Markers,* July–Sept. 1989; 4 (3): 157–62.
7. Blask, D. E., and A. M. Lemus-Wilson. Breast cancer: a model system for studying the neuroendocrine role of pineal melatonin in oncology. *Biochem. Soc. Trans.,* May 1992; 20 (2): 309–11.
8. Mocchegiani, E., N. Fabris, et al. The zinc-melatonin interrelationship. In *Annals of the New York Academy of Sciences,* vol. 719, May 31, 1994; 298–307.
9. Barni, S., P. Lissoni, M. Cazzangia, A. Ardizzoia, F. Paolorossi, F. Brivio, M. Perego, G. Tancini, A. Conti, and G. Maestroni. Neuroimmunotherapy with subcutaneous low-dose interleuken-2 and the pineal hormone melatonin as a second-line treatment in metastatic colorectal carcinoma. *Tumori,* 1992; 78 (6):383–87.
10. Lissoni, P., G. J. Maestroni, et al. Immunological effects of a single evening subcutaneous injection of low-dose interleuken-2 in association with the pineal hormone melatonin in advanced cancer patients. *J. Biol. Regul. Homeost. Agents,* 1992; 6 (4):132–36.

Chapter 29

DHEA

We have, after much study and deliberation, finally decided to go on dehydroepiandrosterone (DHEA) replacement therapy. Eberhard is taking 50 mg and Phyllis 25 mg of micronized (finely powdered) DHEA.*

We take our DHEA after breakfast, together with all our morning antioxidants (see Chapter 11). At the same time, we are also taking 1 tablespoon of flaxseed oil and ¼ teaspoon of borage oil. The antioxidants serve the double purpose of preventing the peroxidation of both the oils, as well as of the DHEA.

*Thus far, we have found only one source for nonprescription micronized DHEA—the Life Extension Foundation (1-800-544-4440). Otherwise, you have to get a prescription and order your DHEA from either one of the following compounding pharmacies: Bellmar Pharmacy (1-800-525-9473), or Women's International Pharmacy (1-800-279-5708).

The decision to add DHEA to our daily health-protective program was not easy. Like melatonin, DHEA is a hormone—a steroidal hormone, in fact, and considered one of our "master hormones" (along with the pituitary gland). It affects every other hormone of the endocrine (hormonal) system, notably estrogen and testosterone. Although these sex hormones are mainly produced by the ovaries and testicles, the body can also convert DHEA into estrogen and testosterone, which has, as we shall see, many implications with respect to DHEA replacement therapy. One obviously does not want to play around blithely with such a powerful hormone.

But first, how do our bodies produce DHEA and how does it work?

DHEA is produced by the adrenal glands that sit atop the kidneys. However, when one is taking oral DHEA, the liver will metabolize most of it to its sulfated form DHEA-S, and only a small fraction of it will appear in the blood as DHEA.[1] Large amounts of DHEA-S are also made in the brain and the peripheral nervous system. That's why its French discoverer, Dr. Etienne-Emile Beaulieu (who also discovered the controversial "morning-after" pill RU 486), calls the sulfated form of DHEA a "neurosteroid." But although the two forms of this hormone are chemically very similar, the way they act in the body are quite different.

Put briefly, DHEA-S seems to be the active form in the brain, while DHEA is active in the rest of the body. But it is difficult to separate the functions of DHEA from those of DHEA-S. We shall therefore refer to DHEA here only as meaning the combined effects of these, for all practical purposes, inseparable twin hormones.

Mental/Psychological Effects

Several animal studies refer to marked memory and learning improvement with DHEA administration.[2] Thus far, at least one detailed human case study has shown a significant improvement in short-term memory with DHEA supplementation in a forty-two-year-old patient with prior low DHEA levels.[3]

DHEA also modifies aggressive behavior, as studies with mice have demonstrated.[4] One can only hope that subsequent studies will also show this effect in humans!

What DHEA has already shown in humans is that it can produce a marked mood elevating and antidepressant effect. In Europe, where DHEA has been more readily available for some time, it has actually been used for the treatment of postmenopausal depression.[5] The effect is usually expressed by those participating in human studies as "a remarkable increase in perceived physical and psychological well-being,[6] associated with a deeper, more restful sleep."[7]

If such benefits were not enough, there is even a hint that DHEA might protect against Alzheimer's disease (DHEA levels have been found to be low in Alzheimer's patients).[8] If so, this would indeed be a blessing, since there is at present no known treatment for the prevention or cure of this dreadful, progressive disease, which slowly destroys the cognitive parts of the brain needed for intellectual functioning.

Physiological Effects

It has been assumed that DHEA exerts a strong protective effect against heart disease—at least, for men. (No such advantage has, until now, been seen for women. In fact, high DHEA levels are thought to put women—particularly postmenopausal women—at greater risk.[9]) Researcher Elizabeth Barrett-Connor, M.D., found that DHEA protected the heart less than had been thought. But she still believes that DHEA provides some protection against not only death from cardiovascular disease, but death from all causes. She also expects final research results to show that men and women are, in fact, equally protected by DHEA against cardiovascular disease.[10]

There is, however, little doubt that DHEA protects against coronary artery disease (atherosclerosis) in many direct and indirect ways. Cardiologist Dr. David Herrington found a statistically significant trend for less and less coronary artery disease with rising DHEA levels. He also confirmed earlier reports by other researchers that DHEA is useful in heart transplants. His five-year survival data showed that patients naturally high in DHEA had an 87% survival rate, whereas those low in DHEA had only a 65% survival rate.[11]

These findings suggest that DHEA supplementation might result in still more favorable outcomes. Other researchers demonstrated (in animal experiments) that dietary DHEA can prevent the rapid development of atherosclerosis that typically follows heart transplants.[12]

There is also a great deal of indirect experimental evidence for DHEA's effectiveness against cardiovascular disease. As is well known, platelet aggregation (clot formation) in arteries can lead to heart attacks or strokes. In one experiment, cardiologist Robert L. Jesse, M.D., put a clot-promoting substance (arachidonic acid) into the bloodstream of ten healthy male volunteers aged twenty-five to thirty-five, then gave them DHEA, and later on collected their blood to check for platelet aggregation (the first step in the formation of atherosclerotic plaque). The DHEA not only slowed platelet aggregation, it virtually prevented clotting.[13]

Dr. Jesse also found that when he gave rabbits DHEA, then damaged the insides of their arteries with a balloon (as is done in angioplasty to open up clogged blood vessels in humans), only 25–28% of them developed restenosis (the clogging up again of the opened blood vessels). In contrast, the blood vessels of rabbits not given DHEA clogged up again in 68% of cases.[14]

Other benefits of DHEA include the following preventive or therapeutic properties:

- helps control insulin levels in diabetes[15]
- helps stop loss of bone mass and demineralization (osteoporosis)*[16]
- lowers high blood pressure (hypertension)[17]
- lowers triglycerides (but apparently not cholesterol, or only slightly)[18]
- is preventive and therapeutic with autoimmune diseases like arthritis, rheumatoid arthritis, systemic lupus erythematosus, and possibly even chronic fatigue syndrome[19]
- makes the immune system more efficient, for instance, by stimulating helper T cells to produce more interleukin-2 (a vital part of the immune system),[20] and in several other ways.[21]
- has anticancer effects.[22]

DHEA even protects against "acute lethal viral infections"[23] and one study showed that *Cryptosporidium parvum* infection was inhibited by DHEA treatment.[24] This is of special importance for AIDS patients, many of whom succumb to the lethal diarrhea caused by this intestinal infection.

Some scientists think that "the salutary immune changes [caused by DHEA] could account for the clinical and experimental evidence of antioncogenic [anticancer] effects of this steroid."[25] There is, for instance, considerable scientific evidence from animal studies that DHEA treatment may inhibit spontaneous breast cancer and lymphoma, as well as a number of artificially induced cancers, such as lung tumors, colon tumors, testicular tumors, prostate cancer, and certain blood-

*A recent study found that DHEA-S levels are "significantly lower" in postmenopausal women with osteoporosis. Since this does not appear to be an effect of differing estrogen levels between women with or without osteoporosis, the researcher concluded that the difference is due to differing DHEA-S levels in these two groups. Miklos, S. Dehydroepiandrosterone sulphate in the diagnosis of osteoporosis. *Acta Bio-Medica del Ateneo Parmense,* 1995; 66 (3–4): 139–46.

borne cancers (hemangiosarcomas). [26] One study also found that increasing serum levels of DHEA in rats to levels comparable to those of adult women reduced the incidence of deliberately induced malignant breast tumors from 68 to 16.5%. All of this was reassuring to us, since concerns about possible cancer risk had made us, up to now, hesitant about DHEA replacement.

In a very different area of human physiology, DHEA is reputed to prevent pyorrhea (bleeding gums). This may sound trivial to some, but is of considerable interest to people like us, who have had gum surgery as a consequence of this age-related and difficult-to-control disease. (CoQ-10 also helps to prevent it.) Anything that holds promise of preventing as odious an affliction as this is surely more than welcome.

DHEA is also known to counteract obesity in postmenopausal women; but this does not constitute, in our opinion, sufficient reason for taking it. Much more important are findings that people on DHEA replacement experience an increased sense of well-being and more energy, are better able to handle stress, and, in some cases, have noticed "marked improvements of preexisting joint pains and mobility."[27]

Sound like claims on a bottle of "snake oil" from the 1800s? Maybe it does. But every one of these claims is backed up either by scientific experiments (the reason for our copious bibliographic references), or by clinical experience. Meanwhile more and more research keeps piling up, confirming the earlier studies about DHEA's effectiveness in all these areas. Besides, we can confirm some of these effects from our own experience, especially with regard to DHEA's mood-elevating effect, which both of us noted within a few days of DHEA replacement therapy.

But why is it that so many of us—especially people over fifty, but some younger ones, too—need DHEA replacement? Just as is true for other hormones like estrogen and testosterone, thymosin, and melatonin, our bodies produce enough DHEA during our youthful years, but less and less with advancing age. In fact, by the time we are seventy, serum DHEA and DHEA-S are about 20% of their peaks between the ages of twenty and thirty. By the age of ninety, only 5% is still circulating in the body.[28]

In addition, some people's bodies don't seem to produce enough DHEA, at any age. This may, in large measure, account for the high incidence of breast cancer in premenopausal women with low DHEA levels. Using supplements to bring lower-than-normal DHEA levels up to where they should be, no matter your age, does therefore make sense. (We think every premenopausal woman with breast cancer in her family history should have her DHEA/DHEA-S levels checked.)

In our own case, tests showed that both of us were, as expected for our ages, low in both forms of DHEA, with Eberhard being extremely low. Also, the above-mentioned benefits of DHEA sounded very attractive to us because—despite our health-protective diet and antioxidant program—we both, to be perfectly honest, still feel the effects of aging. Yet, to repeat, before starting DHEA replacement, we wanted to be sure there was no realistic cancer risk involved for either of us. What good is it, if DHEA does all sorts of wonderful things for you, but may also give you cancer?

In Phyllis's case, we had to carefully consider the breast cancer risk. Laboratory experiments with some breast cancer cell lines had discovered the disturbing fact that where estrogen levels are low (as in postmenopausal women) DHEA stimulates tumor growth. (As we shall see, quite the opposite is true for premenopausal women, for whom DHEA exerts an antitumor effect.)[29]

Phyllis was not only postmenopausal but, many years ago—for prophylactic cancer protection—had her ovaries removed in the course of a radical hysterectomy. Moreover, for a number of reasons, she stopped taking estrogen replacement some years ago. What little estrogen she was getting internally was what her adrenal cortex was producing, or what she got from certain foods, for instance, soy foods such as tofu and tempeh. In other words, she was low not only in DHEA but also in estrogen—not a very safe hormonal milieu in which to start DHEA replacement. So the only way she could take DHEA was if she simultaneously went on estrogen replacement so that her estrogen level would resemble more that of a premenopausal woman.

Eberhard, on the other hand, had to think about the possibility of DHEA increasing the statistically high risk for prostate cancer for men in his age group—for men over eighty, it is a shocking 80%. Frequently autopsies of older men who have died of causes other than prostate cancer reveal that they had prostate cancer as well. Prostate cancer in men of Eberhard's age, in other words, is almost universal. Taking anything—especially a hormonal steroid—that might increase this already high risk would therefore have to be considered carefully.

Our comprehensive literature search in this area revealed a contradictory and confusing picture. On the one hand, there is indeed evidence from a few experiments with mice and rats, and from a laboratory study with a prostate cancer cell line, in which DHEA encouraged malignant prostatic cell growth.[30] There is also the well-known fact that prostate cancer is associated with high levels of testosterone, especially with its active metabolite, dihydrotestosterone, which stimulates both normal and cancerous prostatic cell growth.

Furthermore, as already pointed out, DHEA is a substrate or forerunner of these sex hormones. In fact, certain prostate cancer therapies aim at blocking the production not only of testosterone, but of DHEA-S as well. All of this must be worrisome to any man contemplating DHEA replacement.

On the other hand, there is, as we have seen, also considerable evidence of DHEA's anticancer and immune-boosting effects, against both cancer in general and with regard to prostate cancer in particular. First of all, men with prostate cancer typically have higher testosterone levels and lower DHEA levels than other men. In other words, there is no one-to-one relationship between DHEA levels and testosterone levels. As one group of researchers reported, "We found significantly lower DHEA levels in patients with prostatic cancer and heart diseases."[31]

Another group of researchers put it this way: "It seems

unlikely that serum levels of DHEA or DHEA-S are important risk factors for prostate cancer."[32] And two prominent DHEA researchers (Regelson and Kalimi) report: "We looked for, but did not see, an effect [of DHEA] on prostate growth."[33]

Even more reassuring to us was a study in which human prostatic cancer was transplanted into mice. The mice were then fed DHEA, mixed in with their regular chow. Even in the presence of human prostate cancer cells in these animals, DHEA did not cause tumor growth.[34]

Eberhard seemed to be even less at risk than many other men, for he was very low not only in DHEA but also in testosterone. Even if, as expected, DHEA supplements brought his male sex hormones back to normal levels, this was not likely to pose a serious risk. Even so, Eberhard consulted our good friend and his doctor, oncologist Dr. Robert Nagourney, and only after getting the green light from him did he go on DHEA replacement therapy.

In fact, we might have worried too much. DHEA seems, overall, to *protect* against cancers. In one experiment, for instance, fifteen young male rats of a strain that is very prone to testicular cancer were fed a diet containing DHEA, while a control group of matched rats received normal rat chow. At the end of the experiment (which took the rats to what is "old age"), none of the fifteen DHEA-supplemented rats had developed testicular tumors, while most of the others had.[35]

As far as breast cancer and DHEA is concerned, the existing animal research is also encouraging. For instance, in a strain of mice that spontaneously develops breast cancer, long-term supplementation with DHEA was found to be protective.[36]

Another mouse study, this one on colon cancer, was particularly interesting to us because of Eberhard's history with a precancerous colon tumor. It found that DHEA delayed the appearance of deliberately induced colon tumors.[37]

Still another mouse study found that DHEA inhibits the growth of melanoma cells and encourages normal cell differentiation. This is also of considerable personal interest to Eberhard, who has had two small melanoma lesions (a very dangerous, highly metastatic type of skin cancer)* surgically removed.[38]

As for DHEA and liver cancer, one study found that DHEA inhibited the development of liver cancer in rats treated with chemical carcinogens.[39] Soon after this happy discovery, however, it transpired that there was also a downside with regard to DHEA's long-term effects on the liver. The bad news is that DHEA mimics the toxic effects of certain chemicals on a type of microscopically small organs within liver and kidney cells. This can lead to liver enlargement and, paradoxically—since DHEA is basically a cancer preventor—even to the development of liver cancer. (At least it did so in rats, which do, however, metabolize DHEA very differently from us humans.)[40]

At the root of this seeming paradox seems to be that it is not DHEA, per se, that is responsible, but incidental oxidative stress and oxidative DNA damage.[41] In that case, the good news is that we should be able to prevent oxidative stress by the simultaneous use of antioxidants and therby avoid these unwelcome side effects.

There is still another precaution that we consider essential for maximizing the benefits of DHEA replacement and minimizing its possible risks, especially with regard to possible liver damage and liver cancer: take it together with a little flaxseed oil or borage oil, as we do. (As we said before, it is also a good precaution to take some antioxidants at the same time as taking DHEA.)

*Melanoma is not only the most malignant of all skin cancers, but is considered among the most malignant of *all* cancers. It can rapidly spread to other organs and tissues in the body, including the brain and the spinal cord. However, if detected in the early stages, before it has reached the lymphatic and blood vessels in the second level of the skin (the dermis), it is often curable by limited surgery. (Malin Dollinger, M.D., et al. *Everyone's Guide to Cancer Therapy*. Kansas City: Andrews McMeel, 1991).

For better and faster absorption of DHEA use only micronized (finely pulverized) DHEA rather than the more coarsely milled type, which is unfortunately the kind used in most DHEA products.

Wrapping Up: DHEA and Breast Cancer

The effect of DHEA on premenopausal women is very different from that on postmenopausal women. In premenopausal women, estrogen levels are normally high and androgen (male hormone) levels low. However, low DHEA levels in premenopausal women mean increased breast cancer risk.[42] We therefore advise premenopausal women to have their DHEA level checked and discuss DHEA replacement therapy with a nutrition-oriented internist or gynecologist.

Postmenopausal women, on the other hand, with low estrogen and low DHEA levels should, theoretically, benefit from DHEA supplementation, including cancer protection.

Inversely, high DHEA levels and low estrogen levels might put postmenopausal women at increased breast cancer risk.[43] In this case, DHEA raises androgen (male hormone) levels, without enough counterbalancing estrogens (as in premenopausal women). The DHEA then competes with the sparse estrogen for its receptors on cells, thereby encouraging the growth of breast cancer cells. (For that reason, Phyllis is taking simultaneous estrogen and DHEA replacement therapy.)*

Correct dosage is, however, especially important for postmenopausal women. The protocols in most DHEA studies with postmenopausal women have called for daily doses of 50 and

*We prefer natural estrogens (including estradiol, estriol, and estrone) and natural progesterone, as supplied by, for instance, the International Women's Pharmacy (1-800-279-5708). Ask for their free information kit and a list of prescribing specialists in your area.

100 mg.[44] A recent study, however, found that even 50 mg of DHEA per day "may be excessive" for women, resulting in "supraphysiological" levels that may cause sleeplessness and agitation.[45] The researchers therefore suggested a lower dose of perhaps 25 mg per day for postmenopausal women (exactly the dose Phyllis is taking).

The Bottom Line on DHEA

Here is how internationally famous endocrinologist Dr. Samuel Yen, of the University of California in San Diego, and two other famous DHEA specialists, put it in a recent paper:

> DHEA in appropriate replacement doses appears to have remedial effects with respect to its ability to induce an anabolic growth factor, increase muscle strength and lean body mass, activate immune function, and enhance quality of life in aging men and women, with no significant adverse effects." (Samuel S. C. Yen, A. J. Morales, and O. Khorram, "Replacement of DHEA in Aging Men and Women—Potential Remedial Effects." In *Annals of the New York Academy of Sciences, vol. 774, Dec. 29, 1995, 140).*

Another well-known medical DHEA expert, Dr. Maria D. Majewska, of the Medications Development Division, National Institute on Drug Abuse, Rockville, Maryland, made the following statement: "A few controlled studies and a wealth of anecdotal evidence indicate that DHEA treatment in aging patients is both safe and beneficial." Maria D. Majewska, "Neuronal Actions of Dehydroepiandrosterone," in *Annals of the New York Academy of Sciences,* vol. 774, Dec. 29, 1995, 116.

With regard to the safety of DHEA, the earlier cited Dr. Yen, in answer to a question about side effects, could think only of the possibility that—if used in excessive doses—it may produce acne, masculine hair growth and a malelike, receding hairline in women. In men it can, under these circumstances, result in higher estrogen production (feminizing effect).

None of this will, of course, happen if correct replacement doses are used. Dr. Yen obviously is not worried—he is taking DHEA himself!

Another famous DHEA expert, seventy-year-old William Regelson, M.D. (*The Superhormone Promise*), told writer Gail Sheehy, "I can't wait thirty more years for the National Institute on Aging and [more] double-blind studies [on DHEA] . . ."* He, too, is taking DHEA.

Our Own Experience with DHEA

The tangible beneficial effects of DHEA seem to have been most obvious with Eberhard. Perhaps this is because of his more advanced age and because his DHEA was much more depleted than that of Phyllis.

Most noticeable are, no doubt, the much greater energy and dramatic mood improvement. (Perhaps this comes under the heading of the "remarkable sense of well-being" which people on DHEA therapy have been reporting in several of the earlier mentioned studies.) Frankly, that alone would, for us, be reason enough to be taking DHEA.

What we don't understand is that the participants in some studies with DHEA replacement therapy reported "no improvement in libido." To us, this is almost incomprehensible: a dramatic surge in libido (meaning greater sex interest, sex feelings, and physical manifestations, such as nocturnal and morning erections with Eberhard) was among the first things we noticed.

This coincides completely with what DHEA researcher, Dr. William Regelson, emphatically told Gail Sheehy in the above-mentioned interview: "When you're over sixty and you wake up in the morning with the flag flying, it comes as a sur-

*Sheehy, G. "Endless Youth." *Vanity Fair,* June 1996.

prise. When I started taking DHEA nine years ago, the change in my libido was striking."

The same thing happened with a patient of ours in his mid-seventies, who had been virtually impotent for some time. A few days after being on DHEA, he excitedly called to give us the happy news that his "flag was flying again, too." Other male patients have since reported similar experiences with DHEA (especially when taken together with yohimbine).

As for Phyllis, she also noticed a decided increase in libido, although her response has been less dramatic, as is true for most women. (Some women, however, report a tremendous increase in sexual feeling and desire.) At any rate, it is difficult to imagine that an increase in the general sense of well-being, as is typical with DHEA, would not also have a positive effect on a person's libido.

NOTES

1. Yen, S. S. C., A. J. Morales, and O. Khorram. Replacement of DHEA in aging men and women—potential remedial effects. In *Annals of the New York Academy of Sciences,* vol. 774, December 29, 1995; 146.
2. Robel, Paul, and E. E. Beaulieu. Dehydroepiandrosterone (DHEA) is a neuroactive steroid. In *Annals of the New York Academy of Sciences,* vol. 774, December 29, 1995; 101.

   Flood, J. F., et al. Age-related decrease of plasma testosterone in SAMP8 mice: replacement improves age-related impairment of learning and memory. *Physiology and Behavior,* April 1995; 57 (4): 669–73.

   Roberts, G. Dehydroepiandrosterone (DHEA) and its sulfate (DHEA-S) as neural facilitators: effects on brain tissue in culture and on memory in young and old mice. A cyclic GMP hypothesis of action of DHEA and DHEA-S in nervous system and other tissues. In M. Kalimi and W. Regelson, eds. NY: Walter de Gruyter, 1990; 13–42.

   Flood, J. F., et al. Memory enhancing effects in male mice of pregnenolone and steroids metabolically derived from it. *Proc. Natl. Acad. Sci. USA* 1992; 89:1567–71.
3. Regelson, W., and M. Kalimi. Dehydroepiandrosterone (DHEA)—the multifunctional steroid. In *Annals of the New York Academy of Sciences,* vol. 774, December 29, 1995; 565.

4. Robel and Beaulieu, *op. cit.,* 103–105.

See also Schlegel, M. L., et al. Studies on the effects of dehydroepiandrosterone and its metabolites on attack by castrated mice on intruders. *Physiol. Behav.,* 1992; 34: 867–70.

Joung, J., et al. Suppressive effects of dehydroepiandrosterone and 3-beta-methyl-androst-5-en-17-one on attack towards lactating female intruders by castrated male mice. II. Brain neurosteroids. *Biochem. Biophys. Res. Commun.,* 174:892–97.

5. Regelson and Kalimi, op. cit., 565. *See also* Murphy, B. E. P. Steroids and depression. *Steroid Biochem. Mol. Biol.,* 1991; 38:537–59.
6. Morales, A. J., and S. S. C. Yen. Effects of replacement dose of dehydroepiandrosterone in men and women of advancing age. *J. Clin. Endocrinol. Metab.,* 1994; 78:1360–67.
7. Ibid., 1363.
8. Leblhuber, F., et al. Age and sex differences of dehydroepiandrosterone sulfate (DHEA-S) and cortisol (CRT) plasma levels in normal controls and Alzheimer's disease. *Psychopharmacology,* 1993; 111 (1):23–26.

Roberts, E., and J. Fitten. Serum steroid levels in two old men with Alzheimer's disease (AD) before, during, and after oral administration of dehydroepiandrosterone (DHEA). In M. Kalimi and W. Regelson, eds. NY: Walter de Gruyter, 1990; 43–46.

9. Ebeling, P., and V. A. Koivisto. Physiological importance of dehydroepiandrosterone. *Lancet,* vol. 343, June 11, 1994; 1479.
10. Report on verbal presentations made at the New York Academy of Sciences' Conference on DHEA, June 1995. In *Life Extension,* vol. 2, no. 3, May 1996; 22–23.
11. Ibid., 23.
12. Nestler, E. J., et al. Dehydroepiandrosterone: The missing link between hyperinsulenemia and atherosclerosis? (Review.) *FASEB Journal,* Sept. 6, 1992; 6(12): 3073–5.
13. Jesse, R., J. Nestler, D. Eich, et al. Dehydroepiandrosterone in vivo and in vitro inhibits platelet aggregation (abstract). *J. Am. Coll. Cardiol.,* 1991; 17:376A.
14. Ibid., 24.
15. Schriock, E. D., J. E. Buster, et al. Divergent correlations of circulating dehydroepiandrosterone sulfate and testosterone with insulin levels and insulin receptor binding. *J. Clin. Endocrinol. Metab.,* 1988; 66: 1329–31.

Schriock, E. D., J. E. Buster, et al. Enhanced post-receptor insulin effects in women following DHEA infusion. *J. Soc. Gynecol. Invest.,* 1994; 1: 74–78.

Nestler, J. E. Regulation of human dehydroepiandrosterone metabolism by insulin. In *Annals of the New York Academy of Sciences,* vol. 774, Dec. 29, 1995; 73–81.

16. Regelson, W., R. Loria, and M. Kalimi. Dehydroepiandrosterone (DHEA)—the "mother steroid" I. Immunolic action. In *Annals of the New York Academy of Sciences,* vol. 774, December 29, 1995; 558.

Spector, T. D., et al. The relationship between sex steroids and bone mineral content in women soon after menopause, *Clin. Endocrinol.,* 1991; 34:37–41.

Taelman, P., et al. Persistence of increased bone resorption and possible role of dehydroepiandrosterone as a bone metabolism determinant in osteoporotic women in late postmenopause. *Maturitas,* 1989; 11:65–73.

Rosenberg, S., et al. Age, steroids and bone mineral content. *Maturitas,* 1990; 12:137–43.

Nordin, B. E. C., et al. The relation between calcium absorption, serum dehydroepiandrosterone, and vertebral mineral density in postmenopausal women.*J. Clin. Endocrinol. Metab.,* 1985; 60:651–57.

Sambrook, P. N., et al. Sex hormone status and osteoporosis in postmenopausal women with rheumatoid arthritis. *Rheum.,* 1988; 31: 973–78.

17. Regelson and Kalimi. DHEA—the multifunctional steroid; op. cit., 567.
18. Casson, P. R., et al. Replacement of dehydroepiandrosterone enhances T-lymphocyte insulin binding in postmenopausal women. *Fertil. Steril.,* 1995; 1029.
19. Sambrook, P. N., et al. op. cit.

Van Vollenhoven, R. F., et al. An open study of dehydroepiandrosterone in systemic lupus erythematosus. *Arthritis Rheum.,* 1994; 37:1305.

Suzuki, T., et al. Low serum levels of dehydroepiandrosterone production by lymphocytes in patients with systemic lupus erythematosus (SLE). *Clin. Exp. Immunol.,* 1994; 99:251.

20. Suzuki, T., et al. Dehydroepiandrosterone enhances IL2 (Interleuken-2) production and cytotoxic effector function of human T cells. *Clin. Immunol. Immunopathol.* 61:202–11.

Yen, S. S. C., A. J. Morales, and O. Khorram. Replacement of DHEA in aging men and women—potential remedial effects. In *Annals of the New York Academy of Sciences,* vol. 774, Dec. 29, 1995; 135.

21. Regelson, et al.; DHEA—the "mother steroid." op. cit., 588.
22. Regelson and Kalimi, DHEA—the multifunction steroid, op. cit., 566.
23. Booster, J. E., et al. Postmenopausal steroid replacement with micronized dehydroepiandrosterone: preliminary oral bioavailability and dose proportionality studies. *Am. J. Obstet. Gynecol.,* 1992; 166:1163–70.
24. Regelson, et al. DHEA—the "mother steroid," op. cit., 556.

25. Casson, P. R., et al. Oral dehydroepiandrosterone in physiologic doses modulates immune function in postmenopausal women. *Am. J. Obst. & Gynecol.,* Dec. 1993; 169 (6):1536–39.
26. Schwartz, A. G., and L. L. Pashko. Method of cancer preventive action of DHEA. In *Annals of the New York Academy of Sciences,* vol. 774, December 29, 1995; 180–85.
27. Morales and Yen, op. cit.
28. Labrie, F., et al. DHEA and peripheral androgen and estrogen formation: intracrinology. In *Annals of the New York Academy of Sciences,* vol. 774, December 29, 1995; 16.

    See also Birkenhager-Gillesse, E. G., J. Derkens, and A. M. Lagaay. Dehydroepiandrosterone sulphate (DHEA-S) in the oldest old, aged 85 and over. *Annals of the New York Academy of Sciences,* May 31, 1994; 719: 543–52.
29. Ebeling, P., and V. A. Koivisto. Physiological importance of dehydroepiandrosterone. *Lancet,* vol. 343, June 11, 1994; 1479–81.
30. Labrie, C., et al. Stimulation of androgen-dependent gene expression by the adrenal precursors dehydroepiandrosterone and androstenedione in the rat ventral prostate. *Endocrinology,* 1989; 124:2745.

    See also Schiller, C. D., et al. A growth-stimulating effect of adrenal androgens on the R3327 Dunning prostatic carcinoma. *Urol. Res.,* 1991; 19:7.
31. Stahl, F., et al. Dehydroepiandrosterone (DHEA) levels in patients with prostatic cancer, heart disease and under surgery stress. *Experimental and Clin. Endocrinol.,* 1992; 99: 68–70.
32. Comstock, G. W., G. B. Gordon, and A.W. Hsing. The relationship of serum dehydroepiandrosterone and its sulfate to subsequent cancer of the prostate. *Cancer Epidemiology, Biomarkers & Prevention,* May–June 1993; 2(3): 219–21.
33. Regelson and Kalimi. DHEA—the multifunctional steroid, op. cit., 567.
34. Van Weerden, W. M., et al. Effect of adrenal androgens on the transplantable human prostate tumor. *Endocrinol.,* 1992; 131:2909–13.
35. Rao, M. S., et al. Inhibition of spontaneous testicular Leydic cell tumor development in F-344 rats by dehydroepiandrosterone. *Cancer Letters,* Aug. 14, 1992; 65(2):123–26.
36. Schwartz, A. G. Inhibition of spontaneous breast cancer formation in female C3H (A vy/a) mice by long-term treatment with dehydroepiandrosterone. *Cancer Res.*, 1979; 39:1129–32.
37. Nyce, J. W., et al. Inhibition of 1.2-dimethylhydrazine-induced colon tumorigenesis in Balb/c mice by dehydroepiandrosterone. *Carcinogenesis,* 1984; 5:57–62.

38. Kawai, S., et al. Dehydroepiandrosterone inhibits B16 mouse melanoma cell growth by induction of differentiation. *Cancer Research,* 1995; 15: 427–32.
39. Mayer, D., et al. Modulation of liver carcinogenesis by dehydroepiandrosterone. In Kalimi, M., and W. Regelson, *The Biological Role of Dehydroepiandrosterone.* NY: Walter de Gruyter, 1990: 361–85.
40. Rao, M. S., et al. Hepatocarcinogenecity of Dehydroepiandrosterone in the rat. *Cancer Research,* May 15, 1992; 52: 2977–79.
41. Ibid., 2977.
42. Arguelles, A. E., et al. Endocrine profiles and breast cancer. *Lancet,* 1973; 1:165–68.
43. Ebeling and Koivisto, op. cit., 1480.
44. Yen, S. S. C., A. J. Morales, and O. Khorram. Replacement of DHEA in aging men and women—potential remedial effects. In *Annals of the New York Academy of Sciences,* vol. 774, December 29, 1995; 128–41.
45. Casson, P. R., et al. Replacement of dehydroepiandrosterone enhances T-lymphocyte and insulin binding in postmenopausal women. *Fertility and Sterility,* vol. 63, no. 5, May 1995; 1027–31.

Chapter 30

PREGNENOLONE

Both of us are suffering from some loss of short-term memory, as is true for most older people. We are therefore also taking 50 mg of pregnenolone—known among other things for its benign effect on short-term memory.*

Some people might say we are overdoing things, since DHEA, even without pregnenolone, also has a positive effect on mental functioning. But we think there are several good reasons for doing so. For one thing, pregnenolone is the "parent hormone" not only of DHEA but also of other hormones, notably estrogen and testosterone. Furthermore, its memory-

*We are taking our pregnenolone, together with DHEA and some flaxseed oil or borage oil, right after breakfast, rather than on an empty stomach, because we are taking these hormones together with acidic antioxidants and vitamins, which could otherwise result in heartburn.

enhancing effect and its boosting of mental functions are its primary or principal effects, whereas they are only incidental with DHEA. There is even the possibility, as some scientists think, that pregnenolone might be protective with regard to Alzheimer's disease.*

True, we had already noticed some memory improvement with taking DHEA, but we wanted even greater improvement—plus possibly additional protection against Alzheimer's disease.

Nor is there any danger of overdosing on DHEA by simultaneously taking pregnenolone. As Dr. William Regelson points out, pregnenolone cannot really raise DHEA levels on its own.[1] As DHEA levels decline with advancing age, so do levels of a certain enzyme that is absolutely necessary to break down pregnenolone into DHEA. So even if we take pregnenolone supplements, we may still not have enough of this enzyme to produce DHEA from it.

It would therefore be a serious mistake to only take the "master hormone," pregnenolone, hoping that it would produce sufficient DHEA. Moreover, taking only pregnenolone, without also taking DHEA, might involve some risk. As Dr. Regelson questions, "If pregnenolone does indeed prime the pump that produces other hormones, might it not also increase the production of corticosteroids [the stress hormones]?" In that case, he says, it would be all the more important to have DHEA blunt their immunosuppressive effects by also taking DHEA.

Finally, a recent study by the National Institutes of Mental Health revealed that people suffering from chronic depression have abnormally low levels of pregnenolone in their brains and spinal cords.[2] The connection with depression is not yet perfectly clear. Some scientists, however, think that too much of the inhibitory neurotransmitter GABA, which slows down neuron activity when our brains become overloaded with stimuli, may produce depression.[3] Pregnenolone, on the other hand,

*In more serious cases of short-term memory loss, we would also recommend taking a standardized extract of gingko biloba. It is one of the best-researched plant remedies and known to increase blood flow—and, hence, oxygen delivery—to the brain.

seems to prevent GABA from having this depressant effect—another incentive for taking it, especially for older people like us, who have a tendency toward depression.

With melatonin, DHEA, and pregnenolone we have added the missing third arm—hormonal replacement therapy—to our antiaging/anticancer strategy, the other two arms being correct diet and broad-spectrum antioxidant therapy.

Only growth hormone may be missing in our antiaging/antcancer program. At the present state of the art, however, the side effects of available growth hormone are so worrisome that—despite its apparently sensational rejuvenating effects—one cannot seriously consider it. (Not to mention cost: a year's therapy runs between $12,000 and $15,000!)

For the time being, we therefore abide by Dr. Regelson's advice: "Frankly, I don't see any point in a healthy forty-, fifty-, or even ninety-year-old spending money on growth hormone and risking the side effects."* Besides, as Dr. Regelson, who is perhaps the world's foremost expert on hormone therapy, points out, "DHEA has many of these same benefits [as growth hormone]."

However, two growth hormone analogs—more precisely "secretagogues" that tell the pituitary master gland to release more growth hormone—are now well into clinical trials.† You can bet that, when they become available and we can afford them, you'll find us among the first in line!

Thymus Hormone Replacement

If you are over forty, as most of our readers probably are, you can be sure that your thymus gland is greatly atrophied and no longer producing much of the hormonelike thymic proteins necessary for the proper functioning of cell-mediated immunity.

*Regelson, W., M. D., and Carol Colman. *The Superhormone Promise*. NY: Simon & Schuster, 1996; 210.

†Two of the pharmaceutical companies involved in developing growth hormone secretagogues are Merck and Wyeth-Ayerst.

Precursor cells of lymphocytes are, as long as we live, continuously produced in the bone marrow, from where they migrate to the thymus gland. They cannot mature, though, and differentiate into functional T-lymphocytes unless the thymic proteins are present to program them into doing so. And that is less and less likely to be the case with advancing age.

There are ways to compensate for that kind of deficit, though. For instance, researcher Dr. Terry Beardsley has developed a new technology to grow thymus cells in the laboratory and isolate thymus protein A from them. This is the thymus fraction that laboratory and animal studies have shown to be indispensable for T-4 lymphocytes to mature and produce interleukin-2, which, in turn, is necessary for the cell-mediated immune response to come into play.

Dr. Beardsley's thymus product is in the form of a freeze-dried powder, to be taken under the tongue, from where it is absorbed into the bloodstream.* Its main advantage is that, while not exactly cheap (a one-month supply costs approximately $55), it is still affordable for many people and apparently quite effective.

There is another thymus product, which has been obtained from fresh animal thymus tissue by a very sophisticated and costly cell fractionation process. Like the above-mentioned freeze-dried product, this one, too, can be taken by putting it under the tongue, but it can also (Swiss Dr. Hans Niehaus–fashion) be used by intramuscular injection.†

While this is a live-cell product and possibly superior to anything else, it is so expensive (approximately $180 for eight vials, lasting for only as many days). But for specific purposes, such as to quickly rebuild a depleted immune system, for instance, during or after life-threatening illness, it might indeed be worthwhile (as is true also of the cheaper, freeze-dried ver-

*Dr. Beardsley's product BioPro, Thymic Protein A, is available from the Life Extension Foundation (1-800–544–4440).

† This thymus product is called CartCell 200, BCU, distributed by Allergy Research Group, San Leandro, California (1-800–545–9960). Being a "live" product, it has to be shipped in dry ice and kept frozen until used.

sion). There are anecdotal reports that both of these products have been able to protect against infections and to maintain the white cell blood count of cancer patients undergoing chemotherapy.

What are we doing about thymus hormone therapy? Frankly, nothing for now, because we simply cannot afford it. If it were otherwise, we would indeed be taking thymus hormone, at least once or twice a year.

These financial realities are all the more painful in light of the fact that atrophy of the thymus may be a crucial factor in nature's "programmed death" scheme for us humans, and realizing that only a small financial elite will be able to benefit from some of the most important life extending technologies like thymus and human growth hormone therapy that are currently being perfected.

Hopefully, some time in the future, all life-extending therapies—including every type of hormone replacement and even genetic engineering—will become financially available to almost everyone. Meanwhile, we shall certainly avail ourselves of as many of the other health-protective strategies as are fortunately within our means.

A Final Word About Our Additional Supplement Program

In case the reader wonders—and many will—how we manage to take so many supplements, we hasten to add that we do not necessarily take all the mentioned supplements all the time. Rather, we "pick and choose" from this large menu—as we said earlier—taking only those supplements that we seem most in need of at the time.

The only part of our whole program that's really etched in stone and from which we never deviate, even for a single day, is our basic antioxidant program (the Performance Packs from Health Maintenance Programs or either the Life Extension Mix from the Life Extension Foundation, or the Extend Core from

Vitamin Research Products.) Many of the other supplements—no matter how desirable and vital—are really frosting on the cake.

NOTES

1. Regelson, W., and C. Colman. *The Superhormone Promise.* NY: Simon & Schuster, 1996:108.
2. Steiger, A., et al. Neurosteroid pregnenolone induces sleep EEG changes in man compatible with inverse agonistic GABA A-receptor modulation. *Brain Res.,* 1993; 615: 267–27411.
3. Roberts, E. Pregnenolone—from Selye to Alzheimer and a model of the pregnenolone sulfate binding site on the GABA A-receptor. *Biochem. Pharmacol.,*1995; 49:1–16.

Part Six

"Friendly" Foods

So many new scientific facts about immunity-boosting foods—as well as health risks posed by other foods—have come to light in recent years that the famous official "food pyramid" already looks like an artifact from the time of Tutankhamen. You certainly won't find sea vegetables or tofu and tempeh on the food pyramid, much less things like whey protein, colostrum, or fructo-oligosaccharides, all of which we shall discuss in the following chapters.

In the first edition of *Formula for Life,* we had, for instance, called attention to the many studies about the health-protective properties of sea vegetables (seaweeds) and urged our readers to use them in their diets. To be quite honest, though, we had not yet fully appreciated just how important it is for your health to complement land vegetables with those of the sea on a regular basis.

Also, despite having previously called attention to the importance of soy beans, as well as soy-based tofu and tempeh for any health-protective diet, we had overlooked the role of miso, made from fermented soy paste—a basic food in Japan, Korea, and parts of China, as well as an important item in macrobiotic diet. Now we understand that miso is highly anticancer and good for the immune system. So by simply adding sea vegetables (seaweeds) to miso soup—something Asian populations have done for centuries—we can enjoy the health benefits (and, we think, nice taste) of both of these foods. (See Chapter 32, " 'Seaweeds': Healing Food from the Sea.")

We also recently added whey protein concentrate to our diet. Whey protein concentrate not only has great nutritional value, but—if specially processed and not "denatured" by too high pasteurization methods, spray drying, etc.—can also be an effective, immunity-boosting food. Actually, its high-protein content alone makes it important for vegans and semivegetarians like ourselves, who do not get much protein from animal sources. Add to that the immunity-enhancing effect of undenatured whey protein, and you have indeed a superfood not only of exceptionally high nutritional but also medicinal value. (See Chapter 40, "Whey Protein: Virtual 'Mother's Milk' for Everyone.")

Soy protein concentrate also is a good source of vegetarian protein and useful for weight control. But it does not have the same direct immunity-boosting effects as undenatured whey protein. Soy concentrate, though, has a high content of the anticancer compound genestein, which recommends it for cancer prevention. On the other hand, since soy products raise estrogen levels, some doctors (for instance, the earlier quoted Dr. Charles Simone) warn women not to overuse soy products.*

Aside from these recent additions, our diet has remained pretty much the same since we wrote the first edition of *Formula*

*We think this warning applies more to premenopausal than to postmenopausal women, who may be taking no estrogen replacement therapy and are using soy protein and/or other plant estrogens in lieu of Premarin and similar pharmaceutical products.

for Life. It is based on grains (primarily brown rice), vegetables, and fruits, with small amounts of fish or scallops (but not shrimp or lobster), and poultry (free-range chicken or turkey), along with still smaller amounts of low-fat cheeses. But more about all that in the chapters that follow.

Chapter 31

Broccoli Sprouts: Power in Smallness

By now everyone knows that eating cruciferous vegetables—cauliflower, broccoli, brussels sprouts, cabbage, kale—protects against heart disease and cancer.[1] The trouble is, they're not favorites with many people. Nor is this surprising: they are gassy and their taste is not to everybody's liking. Moreover, word has got around that you have to eat rather large quantities of them—something like two pounds a week—to get much of a health benefit. That's neither attractive nor feasible for most of us.

All the more welcome is the recent news that—at least as far as broccoli is concerned—all we now have to eat is no more than a little over an ounce of broccoli sprouts to get the same benefits as eating pounds of mature broccoli. The reason is that broccoli sprouts contain from thirty to fifty times the concentration of the protective plant chemicals found in mature broccoli. But to take full advantage of these health protective plant chemicals (so-called isothiocyanates and dithiolthiones)[2] and especially one called sulfurophane,[3] we have to eat them raw, for cooking destroys most of them. Fortunately, eating these raw broccoli sprouts is no problem, for they are rather nice tasting. They actually provide a welcome, tangy flavor to salads, go well with low-fat cream cheese, other cheeses, tomatoes, and many other foods.

The way sulfurophane in broccoli sprouts protects us from various toxic and potentially cancer-causing chemicals and radiation is by mobilizing certain of the body's own detoxifying enzyme systems, such as the important glutathione transferases (see the chapter on glutathione). These enzymes, in turn, operate in cells to break down and eliminate noxious compounds before they do damage to the cell's DNA and set the stage for cancer.[4] In fact, three-day-old broccoli sprouts contain enough sulfurophane and another plant substance called glucoraphanin, as a group of scientists at the Johns Hopkins University School of Medicine in a rat study found to be "highly effective in reducing the incidence, multiplicity, and rate of development of mammary tumors."[5] They therefore concluded that "small quantities of crucifer sprouts may protect against the risk of cancer as effectively as much larger quantities of mature vegetables of the same variety."[6]

Broccoli sprouts are now available in this country in many health food stores and some supermarkets. You can, of course, prepare your own broccoli and cauliflower sprouts from seeds. The only thing one must keep in mind, though, is that the seeds must not have been treated with fungicides and insecticides, which is the case with most commercially available seeds. The alternative is to use these treated seeds to grow your own plants, and then use seeds from them for sprouting.

NOTES

1. Wattenberg. L. W., et al. Dietary constituents altering the responses to chemical carcinogens. *Fed. Proc. Am. Soc. Exp. Biol.*, 1976; 35: 1327.

2. Wattenberg, L. W., and W. D. Loub. Inhibition of polycyclic aromatic hydrocarbon-induced neoplasia by naturally occurring indoles. *Cancer Res.*, 1978; 38: 1410.
3. Ansher, S. S. Biochemical effects of dithiolthiones. *Fed. Chem. Toxicol.*, 1986; 24: 405–415.
4. Wattenberg, L. W. Inhibition of neoplasia by minor dietary constituents. *Cancer Res.* (Supplement), 1983; 42:2448S–53S.
5. Fahey, J. W., Y. Zhang, and P. Talalay. Broccoli sprouts: an exceptionally rich source of inducers of enzymes that protect against chemical carcinogens." *Proc. Natl. Acad. Sci. USA,* vol. 94, September 1997; 10367–72.
6. Ibid.

Chapter 32

"Seaweeds": Healing Food from the Sea

In Japan, China, and Korea, the many varieties of sea vegetables (seaweeds) are an important part of the diet and have been highly esteemed for their medicinal and nutritional qualities throughout history. Americans and Europeans, however, lack the necessary information to motivate them to incorporate these important health foods into their diets.

Yet, ounce for ounce, sea vegetables are at least as high in vitamins, carotenoids, minerals, and trace elements as any land-grown vegetables. Moreover, their minerals, including calcium, are in the most bioavailable form for absorption.

More important yet, red/brown sea vegetables—such as wakame, alaria, and kombu (kelp)—contain a number of complex types of sugars called polysaccharides, which have been shown to be effective against many types of cancer.* Alexandra Dundas Todd, in her touching book *Double Vision,* which recounts her son's recovery from brain cancer by a combination of "mainstream" medical therapies (surgery and radiation) and a macrobiotic diet, cites further evidence of the anticancer effects of these compounds in sea vegetables.[1] She mentions, for example, a Harvard School of Public Health study showing a later onset of induced mammary cancer in rats fed "seaweed" than in those fed on regular chow.[2]

There is also substantial research showing that alginates in brown "seaweeds" are capable of "preventing absorption of radioactive products of atomic fission," as scientists from McGill University in Montreal stated at a medical symposium in 1967.[3] This finding may have something to do with a fascinating story told by Dr. Tatsuichiro Akizuki, head of Internal Medicine at a Nagasaki hospital, at the time of the atomic bomb explosion.

As told by Mrs. Todd in her book, Dr. Akizuki claims he saved his patients and himself from the effects of atomic fallout by following a diet of brown rice, miso soup, and sea vegetables, plus some regular land-grown vegetables.[4]

Likewise, Prof. Kazumitsu Watanabe, a cancer and radiation expert at Hiroshima University's atomic bomb research center, claims that when miso soup is eaten regularly, it seems to protect against the effects of radiation. It is, however, customary in Japan to add sea vegetables to miso soup, rather than eating it as a clear broth. This raises questions whether the credit for the radiation protection should not go at least equally to the sea vegetables—which have been shown to inhibit the absorption of radioactive strontium[5]—rather than to miso alone.

It has also been known since the 1950s that certain other compounds in sea vegetables are natural antibiotics, able to inhibit the growth of several species of gram-positive and gram-negative bacteria, which can produce cancer-causing chemicals

*The most effective anticancer polysaccharides are sodium alginate in the laminaria species, and fucoidan and beta-sitosterol in the red varieties of the porphyra family of seaweeds.

in the intestines.[6] More recently, it became clear that marine algae also contain antiviral compounds that have been shown in test tube experiments to protect against a variety of viruses, including influenza B virus, polio virus, herpes simplex virus, and encephalomyocarditis virus. Again, this antiviral activity of sea vegetables is likely to have a protective effect against virus-related cancers, such as papilloma virus-induced cervical cancer and certain types of leukemia.

In the late 1980s, it also became clear that a particular type of sea vegetable, wakame (*Undaria pinnatifida),* showed anticancer activity. At the time, Japanese scientists credited a certain immune system-boosting compound, fucoidan, in wakame for this effect.[7] Later studies confirmed this antitumor effect, but concluded that it was due not just to one specific compound but to "a variety of components in the [wakame] extract."[8]

There is undoubtedly some overlap between the protective compounds in wakame and those in other species of sea vegeables. In other words, different types of sea vegetables are protective in different ways, just as is true for land vegetables. We therefore always use at least two or three different kinds of sea vegetables—such as alaria, kombu (kelp), wakame, dulse, laver, or hijiki—for our miso soup.*

Perhaps, at first, sea vegetables take getting used to, since they don't really compare to anything familiar to our Western palates. But once you have got used to their delicate and incomparable taste—slightly nutty, mushroomy, salty/sweet—we are quite sure you'll soon come to appreciate sea vegetables as much as we do.

A postscript: we used to buy only Japanese and Korean sea vegetables, till we discovered that there are also excellent American sea vegetables. In fact, American kelp cooks more quickly

*For salads, we find sea parsley to be the most convenient and best tasting marine algae. It is a miniature variety of dulse (*Palmaria palmata*), raised in saltwater tanks, because there is not enough of it around in the open sea. One can use either the beautiful, delicate, magenta-colored little florettes, or the dried and powdered version (Ocean Produce International, 1-800-565-8773).

than its Japanese counterpart (kombu), and one variety, dulse, which we are especially fond of, has no Japanese equivalent. We therefore now use mainly Maine coast sea vegetables, and only occasionally add some Japanese or Korean variety that does not grow in our own waters.*

NOTES

1. Todd, Alexandra D. *Double Vision: An East-West Collaboration for Coping with Cancer.* Hanover, NH: Wesleyan University Press of New England, 1994.
2. Teas, J., M. L. Harbison, and R. S. Gelman. Dietary seaweed and mammary carcinogenesis in rats. *Cancer Research,* 1984; 44: 2758–61.
3. Tanaka, Y., D. Waldron-Edward, and S. C. Skoryna. Studies on inhibition of intestinal absorption of radioactive strontium: VII. Relationship of biological activity to chemical composition of alginates obtained from North American seaweeds. *Canad. Med. Assn. J.,* vol. 99. July 27, 1968.
4. Todd, op. cit., 77–78.
5. Tanaka, Y., et al., op. cit.
6. Mautner, G. G., G. M. Gardner, and R. Pratt. Antibiotic activity of seaweed extracts. *J. Am. Pharm. Assn.,* 1953; 42: 294–296.

   Pratt, R., et al. Reports on antibiotic activity of seaweed extracts. *J. Am. Pharm. Assn.,* 1951; 40: 575–579.

   Vacca, D. D., and R. A. Walsh. The antibacterial activity of an extract obtained from *Ascophyllum nodosum. J. Am. Pharm. Assn.,* 1954; 43:24–26.
7. Yamamoto, I., et al. The effect of dietary seaweeds on 7, 12-dimethylbenz (a) anthracene-induced mammary tumorigenesis in rats. *Cancer Lett.,* 1987; 35:109–118.
8. Ohigashi, H., et al. Possible anti-tumor promoting properties of marine algae and *in vivo* activity of *wakame* seaweed extract. *Biosci. Biotech. Biochem.;* 56 (6): 994–995.

*Sea vegetables (seaweeds) are available from health food stores. We buy ours in bulk directly from Maine Coast Sea Vegetables, Franklin, Maine (1-207-565-2907).

Chapter 33

Carotenoid-Rich Vegetables and Fruits

We all know that vegetables and fruits are rich in vitamins and minerals. It is less well known that they also contain many other nutritional and medicinal compounds, such as bioflavonoids, chlorophyll, protease inhibitors, proanthocyanidins (a particularly important type of bioflavonoid), glutathione (a cystein-containing peptide and potent anticancer nutrient), as well as beta-carotene, lycopene, and less well-known carotenoids.

All these natural compounds are represented to a greater or lesser extent in different fruits and vegetables. It is therefore important to eat as large a variety of them as possible to get their full health benefits (just as it is important to take a wide spectrum of antioxidants and other protective supplements to benefit from their synergistic effects).

Carrots and Carrot Juice

Because carrots are so rich in many health-protective compounds, we eat them almost daily, either raw and grated in salads, or lightly cooked. We also highly recommend freshly prepared carrot juice. Not only is it great tasting and refreshing, but it has recently been found to protect against DNA damage in mice, if given immediately after exposure to a chemical capable of causing disruption or breaks in chromosomes, which is the first step in the initiation of cancer.[1]

This protective effect was especially strong if the mice were given an additional drink of carrot juice a couple of hours before exposure to a mutation-causing substance. (The same effect would be achieved, in the human case, by drinking carrot juice regularly.)

Other Carotene-Rich Vegetables

Other favorites of ours that are rich in beta-carotene and similar beta-carotene-like compounds (carotenoids) are spinach, sweet potatoes, broccoli, lettuce, and tomatoes.

We also eat a fair amount of red and yellow bell peppers, both of which have a lot of beta-carotene, as well as other carotenoids (not to mention some of the other, above-mentioned compounds). That is why it is so important not to rely on single supplements, like beta-carotene, but also to eat plenty of the natural foods that contain these other complementary micronutrients.

Significant amounts of carotenoids are also present in some vegetables whose red color is covered up by green chlorophyll. Green bell peppers, for instance, are almost as rich in beta-carotene as their red and yellow varieties. They are also rich in the carotenoids capsanthin and capsorubin,[2] which are probably even more protective than beta-carotene itself.

The same is true for all of the dark green, leafy vegetables.

Of course, the red and brown sea vegetables, like dulse and alaria, also have beta-carotene and many other, related carotenoids.

Tomatoes, too, have some beta-carotene and relatively high amounts of vitamin C, but their glutathione, and particularly their lycopene content, are more important. (See Chapter 7, "Lycopene: The Prostate Saver.")

In addition, tomatoes contain two newly discovered compounds, p-coumaric acid and chlorogenic acid, which are known to block the formation of nitrosamines, found in many processed lunch meats, as well as in cigarette smoke.

Beta-Carotene in Fruits

As in the case of vegetables, yellow/red fruits are also those richest in beta-carotene. That includes, for instance, oranges, cantaloupes, and other yellow melons, as well as watermelons, which, in addition, also have high glutathione content. Tropical fruits like papayas, mangos, and pineapple are also high in beta-carotene and other carotenoids.

NOTES

1. Abraham, S. K., et al. Inhibitory effects of dietary vegetables on the in vivo clastogenicity of cyclophosphamide. *Mutation Res.,* 1986; 172:51–54.
2. Gregory, G. K., et al. Quantitative analysis of carotenoids and carotenoid esters in fruits by HPLC: red bell peppers. *J. Food Sci.,* 1987; 52:1071–73.

Chapter 34

Glutathione in Fruits and Vegetables

Glutathione—like beta-carotene, lycopene, flavonoids, proanthocyanidins, and other natural, health-protective plant compounds—is not a vitamin proper. Rather, it is a peptide, something close to a hormone. In fact, it is a tripeptide, because it is made up of three molecules, the middle one being the important cysteine, which is essential for the body's ability to produce proteins such as collagen (a connective tissue protein).

Glutathione, as we pointed out in Chapter 9, is a powerful antioxidant, free radical quencher, and detoxifier. It detoxifies, for instance, environmental toxins, such as benzopyrines in cigarette smoke or industrial pollution, formaldehyde gas from composition boards in house trailers and many homes, and mercury, lead, and other toxic metals in drinking water.

In addition, it also reacts with hydroperoxides, whether

from outside sources like dietary oils and fats that have started to turn rancid, or produced by normal, metabolic processes in the body itself.* In either case, glutathione transforms these highly toxic molecules into less toxic compounds that the body can get rid of via the urinary or excretory system. Glutathione is therefore crucial for helping prevent both the initiation and promotion of cancer, caused by toxic chemicals like the ones mentioned above and many more.

As to its presence in foods, the sad truth for vegetarians and semivegetarians like ourselves is that there is much less glutathione in vegetables and fruits than there is in meat—for the simple reason that it is present in the highest concentrations in red blood cells.

Nevertheless, there are respectable amounts of it in a number of vegetables and fruits as well. Vegetables highest in glutathione content are, in order of amount, avocados, asparagus, potatoes, okra, and tomatoes; fruits (in usual portion size) are watermelon, grapefruit, strawberries,† oranges, and cantaloupe.

On the other hand, there are fruits, like blueberries and blackberries, that have no glutathione, while most other fruits and vegetables have only trace amounts.‡ It is therefore another instance where—at least for those of us who are not meat-eaters—taking at least an additional 100 mg of glutathione in supplement form is a good idea.

*Toxic formaldehyde is continuously produced in our own bodies during the normal process of cellular metabolism (the chemical processes in the cells that produce energy). There is no way of avoiding it, short of ceasing to breathe and eat. For that reason, an equally continuous process of detoxification, as provided by the body's antioxidants like glutathione and its enzyme systems, has to be in place.

†Strawberries, unfortunately, have the highest pesticide content among fruits. It is therefore advisable to eat, whenever available, only organically grown strawberries.

‡Dr. Dean Jones and co-workers at Emory University have researched the glutathione content of about forty different foods; our summary is based on their findings.

Chapter 35

The Humble Bean Family

When it comes to foods, the old adage "You get what you pay for" just doesn't hold; some of the most nutritious foods are also the cheapest. That's especially true for the family of legumes—beans, peas, lentils, and garbanzos (chick peas). For one thing, their concentration of protein is several times that in cereal grains like wheat, rye, barley, and oats.

Legumes are also a great source of soluble fiber, more precisely, water-soluble gums, which serve several useful functions in the body. They act somewhat like the pectin from fruits by slowing down food absorption (especially important for diabetics). In addition, they inhibit the formation of bile acids, which is protective against colon cancer. This gumlike fiber also seems to be responsible for lowering cholesterol and triglycerides (an effect that is especially pronounced with garbanzos).

Another protective compound in legumes, phytic acid, is

an inhibitor of the destructive hydroxyl radical.[1] Aside from that, legumes also contain protease inhibitors, which laboratory experiments have shown to protect against skin, breast, and liver cancers.[2] (Protease inhibitors are compounds that prevent the enzyme protease from breaking down proteins for digestion. Somehow, this negative effect works, by complicated physiological mechanisms, against tumor formation.)

Many people recognize the high nutritional value and anticancer activity of legumes and even like their taste, but have too much of a problem with their gassiness. That, unfortunately, includes ourselves. But then we read in Mrs. Todd's previously mentioned book, *Double Vision,* how, in her efforts to provide the right kind of nutrition for her son when he was recovering from brain tumor surgery, she discovered that cooking beans together with some kombu (kelp), reduces intestinal gas. We have recently tried this trick, and it definitely helps.

Of course, for digestive purposes, one should always soak beans overnight and discard the water. Beans should then be cooked for a few minutes in new water, and that water must also be discarded. Only then are beans ready to be cooked until done.

Even so, people can have digestive problems with legumes, especially with the most commonly used red and black beans. Rather than avoiding them and thus losing their nutritional benefits, we suggest using a digestive enzyme supplement. On our travels in India, we learned that using a powder containing asafoetida, a natural enzyme that breaks down the troublesome compounds in beans, makes them more easily digestible. (Most Indian stores in America carry such products under different brand names.)

NOTES

1. Graf, E., et al. Phytic acid, a natural antioxidant. *J. Biol. Chem.,* 1987; 262:11647–50.
2. Goldstein, B. D., et al. Protease inhibitors antagonize the activation of polymorphonuclear leucocyte oxygen consumption. *Biochem. Biophys. Res. Comm.,* 1979; 88:854–860.

Chapter 36

Cereal Grains, Nuts, and Seeds

Speaking for ourselves, we never tire of eating many varieties of grains and seeds because we use them in all kinds of combinations with our breakfast cereal, and frequently for lunch and dinner, with other foods. We eat nuts only in season, though, fearing that otherwise their oils might be oxidized and replete with free radicals.

As far as the nutritional value of grains, nuts, and seeds is concerned, it is well established that populations whose diets are predominantly grain-based—such as the Tarahumara Indians of northern Mexico, or the Hunzas of India—are also among the healthiest and live the longest. And for good reason: cereal grains have the highest concentration of complex carbohydrates and fiber. So, while complex carbohydrates provide nature's best fuel for energy, their high fiber content provides for more rapid, intestinal food transport and prompt elimination—a big protective factor, especially with regard to colon cancer.

Michio Kushi and Martha C. Cottrell, the two leading nutritionists of the macrobiotic movement in America, have called attention to the fact that the carbohydrates in cereal grains combine with other nutrients to form certain compounds called glycosaminoglycans that help in detoxifying harmful substances in the body.* (This is also the case with the antioxidant glutathione, which has detoxifying capacity, but which we get very little of from our semivegetarian diet and which, therefore, ranks high on our supplement program—300 to 800 mg a day despite its relatively high cost.)

More important yet, cereal grains, seeds, and nuts are the richest sources of natural vitamin E, another key antioxidant and free radical scavenger. But seeds and nuts have to be fresh, or their vitamin E, which is an oil-like (lipid) substance, is likely to have gone rancid and turned from an antioxidant into a pro-oxidant.

*Kushi, M., and M. C. Cottrell, with M. N. Mead. *AIDS, Macrobiotics and Natural Immunity*. Tokyo and NY: Japan Publications, 1990.

Chapter 37

TOFU AND TEMPEH: HEALTHY ALTERNATIVES TO STEAK AND HAMBURGERS

While many people have trouble digesting beans, including soybeans, fortunately most people have no problem digesting naturally processed soy products, such as tofu* and tempeh,† as well as miso (fermented soy paste). That way, anyone can benefit from the well-documented anticancer com-

*Tofu is made from soybean curd, water, and nigari, a natural sea salt coagulant. It has no fiber whatsoever, but is high in protein. Also, its calcium is said to be very bioavailable (Kushi and Cottrell). We use it mainly in soups (including miso soup) and with vegetable dishes.

†Tempeh is pressed soybean cake, made from split soybeans, water, grains, and special bacterial cultures to produce the desired fermentation. Like tofu, it is high in protein and one of the few vegetarian sources—together with sea vegetables—of vitamin B-12. If you want to raise the already high protein content of tempeh, you may want to try a brand that includes some quinoa, but this advantage is purchased at the price of its characteristic, slightly bitter aftertaste.

pounds in soybeans—unless one is allergic to soy, which is, unfortunately, not as rare as one might think.

Dr. Anne Kennedy of the University of Pennsylvania, one of the country's foremost authorities on the topic, thinks that protease inhibitors, which are bountiful in soy foods, actually "have a selective toxicity for transformed (malignant) cells."[1] If so, Dr. Kennedy says, we may have in these substances "nature's own guided missile system" (similar to radioactive monoclonal antibodies that home in on cancer cells) and can selectively destroy cells with chromosomal abnormalities.

Research by Dr. Kennedy also showed that protease inhibitors in soybean extract are able to suppress oral and rectal cancers in animals, and do so without any untoward side effects. In fact, her studies suggest that these natural substances in soybeans and other legumes might be able to inhibit other cancers as well.[2] If so, these anticancer benefits would, of course, also apply to the fermented soy paste of miso soup.

Dr. Kennedy thinks there is real hope that the cancer-inhibiting effects of these compounds in soybeans and other legumes might apply to cancer not only in animals, but also in humans. She cites, for instance, certain laboratory experiments in which oral cancer was artificially induced in hamsters, but prevented from spreading by protease inhibitors from soybeans. Since these cancers closely resemble human squamous cell carcinoma, the most common form of oral cancer, we may safely assume that soybeans and soy products like tofu, tempeh, and miso also protect against human oral cancers.

Still more anticancer benefits of soy foods have been discovered only recently. Dr. William R. Fair, chief of urology at Memorial Sloan-Kettering Cancer Center in New York City reports that in animal studies, soy protein is almost as protective as a low-fat diet in slowing the progression of prostate cancer.

Nobody should, of course, be tempted to think of substituting tofu and tempeh for a low-fat diet. In fact, tofu and tempeh are relatively high in fat (about 3% saturated fat, 2% polyunsaturated fat, and 1% monounsaturated fat). One should therefore never combine these soy foods with other high-fat foods. For the same reason, it is also not a good idea to fry tofu or tempeh in oils, as often served in Chinese restaurants.

NOTES

1. Kennedy, A., and J. B. Little. Effects of protease inhibitors on radiation transformation in vitro. *Cancer Res.,* 1981; 41:2103–106.
2. Kennedy, A. The condition for the modification of radiation transformation *in vitro* by a tumor promotor and protease inhibitors. *Carcinogenesis,* 1985; 6:1441–45.

Chapter 38

The Incredible Miso Soup

Miso soup, as previously mentioned, is made from concentrated, fermented soybean paste, which comes in various shades, from light ochre to red and dark brown. Each type of miso has a distinct, individual taste. Personally, we like all of them and enjoy changing off between them for variety, or mixing two together.*

We add at least two or three varieties of sea vegetables (seaweeds) and brown rice or whole-grain pasta, and spices to

*When making miso soup, do not expose the miso paste to high temperatures, or the helpful bacteria in it that derive from its fermentation process will be killed. If they are killed by boiling or dissolving the miso in too hot water, you will, of course, still get the benefits of the soya, but not the full medicinal effect of miso containing the live bacteria. In practice, that means adding the miso after the water or the soup has cooled off enough to be eaten.

our miso soup. Frequently, we also add land vegetables, like carrots, broccoli, and zucchini. Other times, we may use azuki beans, soybeans, garbanzos, or lentils. We usually also include tofu (bean curd), or hard-boiled egg whites, fish, or scallops for additional protein. That way we can honestly say that we never get tired of eating miso soup almost daily, and not just because it is probably the best anticancer nutrition there is, but because we really enjoy it.

To our own surprise, miso has recently been reported to contain the compound genistein, which apparently inhibits the blood-vessel growth on which tumors depend.[1] If so, miso soup can play an important supportive role in endostatin and angiostatin therapy. (Shark and bovine cartilage therapy is based on the discovery that cartilage contains certain angiostatic [new blood vessel-inhibiting] and anti-inflammatory compounds, genistein being one of them.)*

We were recently told, on what seems to be reputable (although not yet verified) scientific evidence, that garbanzos also have a mild inhibiting effect on the formation of new blood vessels. In that case, adding garbanzos to miso soup should result in an even greater tumor-inhibiting effect.

It has also been reported by a group of Japanese scientists that in animal experiments, a diet supplemented with miso reduced the incidence and delayed the appearance of artificially induced breast cancer. These scientists therefore concluded that "miso consumption may be a factor producing a lower breast cancer incidence in Japanese women."[2]

As far as sea vegetables are concerned, there is all the more reason—aside from those discussed in our special chapter on them—for their inclusion in miso soup: we are referring to the totally overlooked but possibly very important fact that brown/red sea vegetables have been found, in an obscure and long-forgotten scientific paper, to be capable of "reducing the con-

*As previously noted, though, shark and bovine cartilage are only *mildly* antiangiostatic in comparison to endostatin and angiostatin.

sumption [absorption] of excess sodium," because their calcium alginate supposedly binds to it.[3]

We are not too worried about the salt content of miso, regardless of whether the cited study is correct. As earlier stated, miso contains only unrefined sea salt, which is less objectionable than rock salt, because it also contains potassium, iodine, and other minerals. Also, it has not been chemically treated and bleached. Adding sea vegetables to miso soup raises its potassium and iodine content still further, balancing any additional sodium. We therefore don't hesitate recommending a daily bowl of miso soup with sea vegetables (despite its relatively high sodium content) to anyone, but especially those with cancer or AIDS and others at special health risk.

It is therefore all the more regrettable that Westerners often don't like miso soup—much less miso soup with sea vegetables. Astonishing as it is to us, even a percentage of cancer and AIDS patients—while often getting to like miso soup—can never overcome their dislike of sea vegetables. Fortunately, however, there are even more of those who, like ourselves, become really fond of both miso and sea vegetables, and wouldn't want to be without them.*

NOTES

1. Todd, Alexandra D. *Double Vision: An East-West Collaboration for Coping with Cancer.* Hanover, NH: Wesleyan University Press of New England, 1994; 76.
2. Baggott, J. E., T. Ha, et al. Effects of miso and NaCl on DMBA-induced rat mammary tumors. *Nutrition and Cancer,* vol. 14, 1990.
3. Tanaka, Y., et al. Studies on inhibition of intestinal absorption of radioactive strontium: VII. Relationship of biological activity to chemical composition of alginates obtained from North American seaweeds. *Canad. Med. Assn. J.,* vol. 99, July 27, 1968; 169.

*When preparing miso soup, be sure *not* to use boiling water or add it to other boiling-hot soups. Let the hot water or soup cool off for a few minutes, to approximately 170F° as if you were preparing green tea. Too much heat will kill the helpful miso bacteria. (Remember, miso is made from *fermented* soybeans.)

Chapter 39

Garlic: Nature's Patent Medicine

The use of garlic as a food and medicine goes far back into antiquity. In the Old Testament we read that the Israelites, in their trek through the desert after leaving Egypt, not only lusted after the fleshpots of Egypt, but also missed the garlic they were used to. No wonder onions and garlic found their way into the Talmud and remained stock items in a traditional Jewish diet.

Garlic cultivation, however, did not start in Egypt, although the famous Ebers Papyrus, dating from about 1550 B.C., mentions it as an ingredient in no fewer than twenty two herbal concoctions. Garlic cultivation actually seems to go back, though, to prehistoric times and the Kirgiz desert region of Siberia. From there it apparently migrated eastward to Asia Minor, Egypt, India, and China. So it is not surprising that it figures prominently in traditional Ayurvedic and Chinese herbal medicine. Later, garlic found its way westward to Europe and from there to the Americas.

Garlic's medicinal history includes the names of antiquity's most famous physicians and thinkers. Hippocrates (460–375 B.C.) prescribed garlic for various ills, as did Aristotle (384–322 B.C.), Pliny the Elder (A.D. 23–79), and the Greek physician Galen (f. A.D. 130). Later on, garlic is mentioned by, for instance, the Arab physician Avicenna (980–1037), and William Turner (1510–1568), physician and herbalist to Queen Elizabeth I.

So the humble garlic has a distinguished pedigree, to which we may add none less than Charlemagne, king of the Franks and Emperor of the West (742–814), who praised the healing power of garlic in his own book about medicinal herbs, *Mein Kraeuterbuechlein.* (If you wonder how Charlemagne found time, while conquering the Western world, to think about herbal medicines, so do we.)

Closer to our own times, Louis Pasteur, in 1858, described garlic's antibacterial properties, and Albert Schweitzer used it in Africa to treat amoebic dysentery.

There is now a great deal known about exactly what garlic's medicinal benefits are and how they are achieved. The discussion that follows will therefore be strictly based on the latest and most comprehensive studies.*

According to these scientific sources, garlic seems to have the following medicinal attributes:

- it is antibacterial, antifungal, and antiviral
- it inhibits platelet aggregation (prevents blood clotting)

*Our foremost scientific references for the following discussion are: 1) Dr. Robert Nagourney's excellent review paper, "Garlic: Medicinal Food or Nutritious Medicine?" *Journal of Medicinal Food,* vol. 1, no. 1; 1998; 2) Dr. B. Biederman (Medizinische Klinik, Inselspital, Bern), "Knoblauch: ein geheimstes Wunder Gottes?" ("Garlic: God's Best-Kept Secret?"), *Schweizerische Rundschau für Medicin* (PRAXIS), 84, Nr. 1, 1995; 3) Alexander N. Orekhov (Institute of Experimental Cardiology, Moscow) "Effects of Garlic on Atherosclerosis," and Joerg Gruenwald (Institute for Phytopharmaceuticals, Berlin), *Nutrition,* 1997; vol. 13, nos. 7/8, 656–663.

- it prevents and scavenges free radicals
- it is definitely cancer-preventive

How Does Garlic Work?

Garlic contains several medicinal compounds. Alliin is the primary compound, but alliin must be acted on by a garlic enzyme called alliinase to turn it into allicin, which your body can use. That can happen, though, only when you chop the garlic, or put it through a garlic press, or mash it up some other way, which is necessary to release the enzyme. Of course, just eating raw garlic also releases the enzyme, but few people seem to be that brave!

It is the allicin that gives garlic its characteristic odor and flavor, which some people love and others—at least in our American culture—find so offensive. Elsewhere, though, as in France and Italy—not to mention India and China—garlic is eaten much more regularly and in larger quantities than here and nobody seems to take offense. (It's best that everyone around the table eats garlic and smells the same, so nobody can complain!)

However, while allicin is technically the main active ingredient in garlic, it rather serves as a chemical precursor or forerunner of several other compounds—sulfides and sulfide-containing peptides—that are its most active agents.

Aside from that, garlic also contains carbohydrates, phospholipids, amino acids, glycosides, minerals, vitamins, and the trace elements selenium and tellurium.

Antibacterial, Antifungal, and Antiviral Effects

Extracts of fresh garlic have been found active against fourteen strains of both gram-positive and gram-negative bacteria, including some antibiotic-resistant organisms.[1] Incidentally, the extract of onions, which do *not* contain allicin, is "virtually ineffective" against bacteria—further confirmation that it is the allicin and its breakdown products that are responsible for garlic's antibacterial effect.

It has been discovered, though, that allicin is very unstable when heated. So, if you cook garlic, don't expect any antibacterial effects (and probably no other medicinal effects either), for allicin is deactivated if heated above 133 degrees Fahrenheit (56 degrees Celsius). In other words, if you boil, roast, or fry garlic, all you wind up with is some garlic flavor, but probably no medicinal effects. When you see all those wonderful recipes that involve boiling, roasting, or frying ("glazing") garlic—to make, for instance, different kinds of garlic soup[2]—you now know that you will either have to modify them, or just enjoy them "as is," without kidding yourself that they are going to do much more than just taste good.

Fresh garlic, on the other hand, has been shown to have "significant activity" against several particularly tough and troublesome strains of bacteria, among them *Mycobacterium avium,* isolated from AIDS patients. [3] Garlic has also been found effective (at least, in vitro) against *Pneumocystis carinii,*[4] likewise a frequent complication in AIDS.

This suggests that fresh garlic and certain garlic products—aged garlic, Kyolic garlic, and garlic powder tablets—may be useful in fighting these secondary infections in AIDS patients. This does not mean that garlic or garlic products should replace standard antibiotic therapy, but garlic may enhance the effectiveness of antibiotics.

Equally remarkable is that garlic extract was shown to be effective against the bacterial stomach parasite *Helicobacter pylori,* which has been implicated as frequently being the causative agent in peptic ulcer disease.[5] Here again, garlic, in one form or another—preferably crushed, raw garlic, because of its similarity to the water-extract used in the study—might be useful as an adjunct to standard antibiotic therapy. It might prevent some of the frequent therapeutic failures with antibiotic therapy, and thus make repetitive courses of such therapy, with their often debilitating side effects, unnecessary.

Actually, it is not the allicin in garlic alone that is responsible for this surprisingly powerful antibacterial effect. Rather, ajoene, one of the compounds into which allicin breaks down during digestion, seems to also play a major role. (In that connection, the Spanish name for garlic is *ajo,* obviously deriving from the same Latin root.)

Garlic has also antifungal properties. As Dr. Robert Nagourney points out, several studies show that garlic extract—and, by implication, raw garlic itself—can be as effective as, and in some instances even more effective than, standard antifungal drugs, which, when taken internally, can have unpleasant side effects. Fungus-caused skin problems (like athlete's foot), as well as internal yeast infections—e.g., thrush, a mouth infection caused by *Candida albicans,* and often accompanying AIDS—as well as fungal ear infections, caused by *Aspergillus,* might therefore be treatable with liquid garlic extract, taken internally, as well as applied directly to the affected area. It is certainly worth trying, either alone or in conjunction with standard pharmaceutical products.

As for garlic's antiviral potential, Dr. Nagourney cites recent Chinese studies showing garlic extract's effectiveness against cytomegalovirus (CMV). This discovery led, in turn, to successful trials with garlic extract as prophylaxis against CMV in bone marrow transplant patients.[6] Adjunct therapy with garlic or garlic products thus seems a worthwhile precaution in such cases.

"Broad antiviral activity" of garlic extract has also been reported for test tube experiments against herpes simplex types I and II, vaccinia (a virus that causes cowpox in milk cows and can be transmitted to humans), stomatitis (a viral infection of the mouth with inflammation of the oral mucosa) and, most important, against human rhinoviruses, a class of viruses that cause the common cold.[7] Here, again, fresh garlic (one to three cloves a day), or a standardized garlic product, may be useful, particularly in view of the paucity of pharmaceutical antiviral therapies available.*

We cannot leave this discussion without sharing a European legend with you, meant to illustrate garlic's reputation as a natural antibiotic. As the story goes, in 1721, during a terrible plague in Marseille, four incarcerated thieves were given the chance to pick up and bury the dead. The deal was that if they somehow survived, which nobody expected, they were to go free. But, to everyone's surprise, they survived very well. Their secret turned out to be that they had been drinking a concoction of vinegar with lots of mashed garlic, which, henceforth, became a folk remedy against infections called "vinaigre des quatre voleurs" (four thieves' vinegar).

Garlic for Heart and Circulatory Problems

Let us start with yet another media blitz against a natural remedy, this time concerning garlic. The June 22, 1998, issue of *Time* magazine carried the following item: "Bad News on Garlic: Garlic has been worshiped as a medicinal miracle for centuries, but researchers last week showed that contrary to findings from other studies, garlic-powder supplements do nothing to control cholesterol levels. No significant effect on blood pressure was found either."

This news flash makes it look as if cholesterol and blood pressure control were garlic's main benefits, or even its only ones. Actually, they have always been considered only marginal, albeit previously well-researched benefits of garlic. On the other hand, they have always been overshadowed by its antibiotic and

*We prefer using fresh garlic, but have a high degree of confidence in two garlic products: a standardized garlic extract by Vitamin Research Products (1-800-877-2447), and Pure-Gar caps, also a standardized allicin product, from Prolongevity (1-800-544-4440).

cancer-preventive functions. But few readers will be able to quickly make these mental corrections.

Time magazine does not even take into consideration garlic's effects on several other aspects of cardiovascular health, such as its antithrombotic (blood-clot-preventing), antiarrythmic (irregular heartbeat-preventing), and other antiatherogenic factors that help prevent the clogging of arteries—all of it demonstrated by many excellent studies worldwide.

Instead of presenting a more rounded outlook, the attention-catching news flash (it even featured a photo of a garlic bulb) made it look as if another hoax by the "natural foods crowd" or the health food industry was being exposed. No wonder people are confused and don't know any more who and what to believe.

But let's try to make some kind of sense of it all.

Leaving aside the whole issue of whether garlic does or does not lower cholesterol and blood pressure, its antithrombotic (blood-clot-inhibiting) effect seems to remain unchallenged. There is, for instance, garlic's well-documented capacity to inhibit blood platelet aggregation, as well as its equally well-established ability to inhibit thromboxane formation.[8] (Thromboxane is a prostaglandinlike compound that encourages the clumping together of blood platelets—clot formation—and may result in heart attack or stroke.) In this—thus far, unchallenged—respect, garlic and certain garlic products seem to definitely have potential—as one among many natural products—in helping to prevent heart attack and stroke.

Anticancer Effects

Dr. Junshi Chen, of the Chinese Academy of Preventive Medicine in Beijing—also an expert on green tea (see Chapter 41)—called attention, early on, to the cancer-preventive attributes of garlic, especially with regard to stomach cancer.[9] Nor is this surprising, for the Chinese have had a vivid example of garlic's anticancer effect: they noticed that there is dramatically less stomach cancer among the inhabitants of Gangshang County in Shandong Province. The apparent reason: its people consume, on average, 20 grams of garlic a day (the equivalent of six to seven cloves), much of it, apparently, in raw form. In contrast, the residents of neighboring Qixia, who consume less than 1 gram a day, have astronomically high stomach cancer rates. It was an object lesson that was hard to overlook.[10]

Colon cancer, as one study seems to show, may also be lower in people who consume garlic at least once a week.[11] Another study, though, involving large numbers of men and women in the Netherlands found no such protective effect for breast, colorectal, and lung cancers—at least not when various types of garlic supplements, rather than fresh garlic, were taken. (Different garlic supplements vary so much in effectiveness that one cannot tell much from a study like this. Furthermore, the data for this study were collected by questionnaire, which also casts doubts on its reliability.)

On the other hand, there are intriguing laboratory and animal studies showing how active ingredients in garlic (allicin, ajoene, etc.) might block both initiation and promotion of cancer. This may be caused by garlic compounds binding to carcinogenic substances, inhibiting tumor promotion and mobilizing the body's own protective enzyme systems.

At any rate, as Dr. Nagourney points out, some animal studies have "clearly established the ability of garlic's water-and-lipid-soluble fractions to directly inhibit tumor initiation."[12] Interestingly, though, it turned out that selenium-enriched garlic was more potent in preventing tumor initiation than regular garlic alone. It therefore seems advisable to take a selenium supplement, if garlic is used for cancer prevention. (It is part of our regular additional supplement program.)

As far as skin cancer promotion is concerned, studies have shown that both garlic and onion oils, directly applied to the affected area, inhibit the promotion phase of skin cancer (in animals). Amazingly, test-tube studies with colon cancer cells have even shown that active compounds in garlic are as effective in preventing tumor growth as the chemotherapy drug 5-fluorouracil(5-FU).[13]

Even the optimal dose of garlic for protection against cancer promotion seems to have been determined. Extrapolating from a study on colon cancer in rats, the minimum effective dose for humans seems to be 10 grams a day (three to five cloves). That is obviously more garlic than most people would want to eat. On the other hand, even as little as one large clove a day, which is quite feasible, might be incrementally protective, especially if part of a comprehensive cancer-prevention diet and supplement program.

Finally, garlic's proven ability to inhibit and scavenge free radicals is, by implication, also protective against cancer, for cancers are, at least partially, free radical–driven.

In short, the news about garlic is not as grim as *Time* magazine would have one think, but rather confirms its many medicinal properties, experientially known for several millennia.

NOTES

1. Farbman, K. S., and E. D. Barnett. Antibacterial activity of garlic and onions: a historical perspective (letter). *Pediatric Infect. Disease J.*, 1993; 12(7): 613–14.
2. See, for instance, Barbara Kafka's garlic recipes in *The New York Times*. 24 June 1998.
3. Deshpande, R. G., et al. Inhibition of *Mycobacterium avium* complex isolates from AIDS patients by garlic (*Allium sativum*). *J. Antimicrob. Chemother.*, 1993; 32: 623–26.
4. Abdullah, T. H. In vitro efficacy of a compound derived from garlic against *Pneumocystis carinii* (letter). *J. Natl. Med. Assn.* 1996; 88: 694–704.
5. Cellini, L., et al. Inhibition of *Helicobacter pylori* by garlic extract (*Allium sativum*). *FEMS Immun. Med. Microbiol.*, 1996; 13: 272–77.
6. Lu, D. P. Bone marrow transplantation in the People's Republic of China. Chinese bone marrow transplant registry. *Bone Marrow Transplant*, 1994; 13: 703–704.
7. Weber, N. D., et al. *In vitro* virucidal effects of *Allium sativum* (garlic) extract and compounds. *Planta Medica*, 1992; 58: 417–23.

8. Several references to such studies are cited in Orekhov, A. N., and J. Gruenwald. Effects of garlic on atherosclerosis. *Nutrition*, 1997; vol.13, nos. 7/8; 656–663.
9. Chen, J. The antimutagenic and anticarcinogenic effects of tea, garlic and other natural foods in China: a review. *Biomed. & Environmental Scis.*, 1992; no. 1; 5: 1–17.
10. Mei, X., M. I. Wang, Xu, et al. *Acta Nutrimenta Sinica,* 4: 53–56.
11. Steinmetz, K. A., L. H. Kushi, et al. Vegetables, fruit, and colon cancer in Iowa Women's Health Study. *Am. J. Epidemiol.*, 1994; 139: 1–15.
12. Nagourney, R. Garlic: Medicinal Food or Nutritious Medicine? *J. Medic. Food*, 1998; no.1; 13–28.
13. Sundaram, S. G., and J. A. Milner. Diallyl disulfide inhibits the proliferation of human tumor cells in culture. *Biochem. Biophys. Acta*, 1996: 1315: 15–20.

Chapter 40

Whey Protein: Virtual "Mother's Milk" for Everyone

By lucky coincidence, the composition of whey protein from cow's milk is very similar to that of human breast milk. It is this little-known fact that makes cow whey easily digestible by infants and grown-ups alike. Moreover, it is so similar to human breast milk in its amino acid profile that its nutritional value to us humans is virtually identical.

More remarkable yet, if whey protein has not been "denatured" by high pasteurization temperatures and rough processing methods—that is, if it is in its original, biologically active form—it even has immunity-enhancing properties, almost identical to mother's milk. In other words, specially processed ("undenatured") whey protein—containing biologically active immunoglobulins—can protect us from most of the common infectious diseases of mankind, almost as much so as mother's milk. Too good to be true? Well, we shall show you the research that has been done over the past ten years or so, and you be the judge.

First of all, what is whey? Briefly put, it is the curd-free portion of milk that is left over from the production of cheese.

No more than twenty years ago, whey protein was little more than a nuisance to the cheese industry; nobody knew what to do with it. The only ones interested in it were some smart cattle ranchers who bought it for feed because it was so cheap. The rest was simply thrown away.

Dairy farmers, too, had always known that the whey left over from making cottage cheese was good food for animals and humans. Experience had taught them that when they fed whey to either young calves or their own babies, it made both of them grow and put on weight fast.

Only in recent years has science finally caught up with traditional country wisdom and discovered the many health benefits of whey protein. From there, it didn't take long for modern food technology to concentrate and refine it into water-soluble powders of either whey protein concentrate (WPC), containing 75–85% protein, or whey protein isolate (WPI), containing 90% or more of ultra low-fat whey protein.

Body-builders and athletes were the first to appreciate this new low-fat protein source. They quickly discovered that nearly fat-free whey protein concentrates and isolates made them put on lean muscle mass, while providing them with lots of energy.

But for every body-builder and athlete there are many others who urgently need to regain lost muscle—not to win prizes in muscle shows, or to run the New York marathon, but for sheer survival. A high percentage of AIDS and cancer patients suffer from chronic diarrhea and poor absorption of nutrients. They are in danger of succumbing to the terrible wasting syndrome that is all too often fatal. For them, whey protein concentrates or isolates are the nutritional supplements of choice to help maintain their weight.

Similarly, many of the elderly are malnourished and underweight. They notoriously have little appetite, do not choose the right foods, and do not digest their food properly. They, too, can benefit greatly from a food like whey protein that provides much-needed protein, without burdening their weak digestive systems with hard-to-digest fats and oils, or empty sugar calories.

Paradoxically, WPC or WPI can also be used to lose weight, if combined with a low-calorie diet. It can even be used to replace a meal occasionally. We know, for instance, of some business and professional people who, on especially busy days, make themselves a whey protein drink in the office instead of going out for lunch.

Ironically, though, the problem with available whey protein concentrates and isolates on the health food market is that, because of prevailing processing methods, it is, for all practical purposes, impossible to find one that is not largely denatured and thus no longer biologically active. Not that this makes these products worthless, by any means. They still have high nutritional value and serve, as we shall see, many useful purposes. But if whey protein is to boost our immunity, it must be biologically active (undenatured), and there is, alas, only one product we know of that comes up to these standards.

We shall come back to this important point. First, though, let us talk about the health benefits offered by "regular" whey protein—i.e., whey protein concentrate or isolate that is, to a greater or lesser degree, denatured.

Whey Protein Fights Osteoporosis

Only recently has it been discovered that whey protein concentrate (or isolate) is effective for the prevention and treatment of osteoporosis. One study found that when rats were fed whey protein, they had better bone growth and their bones were stronger than those of rats on regular chow.[1] The researchers concluded that whey protein stimulates both bone cell growth and collagen synthesis. (Collagen is the protein substance of skin, tendon, bone, cartilage, and other connective tissue.)

This stimulating effect on bone cells was present even

when the whey protein was heated for ten minutes between 75 and 90 degrees centigrade (167–194 degrees Fahrenheit), that is, almost to the boiling point.

Since that much heat would obviously denature the whey protein and knock out its immunity-boosting capacity, its ability to foster bone growth and bone density is clearly independent of the degree of denaturation it has undergone. That is good news, if we may extrapolate from the rat study that what is good for rat bones may also be good for human bones, which is not necessarily always the case. But especially if used together with calcium and vitamin D-3 supplements and weight-bearing exercise, chances are that we humans will also reap the bone-strengthening effects of whey protein.

Whey Protein and Cholesterol Control

Whey protein—in contrast to *casein,* a milk protein with cholesterol-*raising* effect—has been shown (again, in a rat study) to have a cholesterol-lowering effect.[2] The study showed that when whey protein concentrate was consumed by these animals, even in relatively small amounts, it reduced liver—though not plasma—cholesterol. The researchers concluded that the mechanism by which this effect was achieved is that "whey protein inhibits cholesterol synthesis [by the liver]."

Even more important, whey protein has also been found (albeit, again, only in animal studies) to prevent the accumulation of oxidized LDL cholesterol in the important white scavenger cells of the immune system called macrophages. When such accumulation is not prevented, these macrophages become precursors of "foam cells," regularly found in early atherosclerotic lesions. Anything to prevent this is therefore more than welcome.

The researchers thought this beneficial effect may be caused by lactoferrin, a substance in whey protein that functions as a natural antibiotic. It tends to enter the space below the inner lining of arteries (the "subendothelial space") and is able to prevent the foam cells from producing the atherosclerotic plaque that clogs up arteries and causes heart attack and stroke.[3]

To repeat: the above-cited health benefits were achieved with whey proteins of unknown quality. They can, therefore, be assumed to have been denatured. Yet they were, as we have seen, able to build lean muscle mass, fight the wasting syndrome that is the bane of AIDS and cancer patients, counteract osteoporosis, help control cholesterol levels, and prevent the buildup of atherosclerotic plaque in arteries. Not a bad scorecard for a single food.

Whey protein concentrate or isolate can, however, achieve even greater health benefits, if special processing methods have been employed to prevent its denaturation and keep it in its biologically active, immunity-boosting state.

Immunity-Boosting Effects of Biologically Active Whey Protein

For a whey protein concentrate (or isolate) to be effective in boosting immunity, it is crucial that the manufacturing process does not damage (degrade) its delicate building blocks, or "whey protein fractions"—beta-lactoglobulin, alpha-lactalbumin, serum albumin, and the immunoglobulins.

That means, above all, lower pasteurization temperatures (or, alternatively, shorter pasteurization time) are critical. In addition, great care has to be taken with regard to certain processing techniques like aeration, vacuum evaporation, and spray drying of the powder. Too much heat, pressure, or agitation will damage these whey protein fractions[4] and thereby diminish their immunity-boosting potential.

If, on the other hand, the whey protein fractions are intact and biologically active, our immune system cells—lymphocytes, natural killer cells, and macrophages—can use them for a very important, immunity-boosting purpose: they can manufacture the important peptide glutathione—a first-class free radical scavenger and detoxifying agent—from some of these sulfide-containing building blocks.

The importance of this becomes instantly clear when we realize that the virus that causes AIDS destroys the patient's T-cells simply by depleting them of glutathione. At the same time, it is extremely difficult—if not, for all practical purposes, impossible—to get glutathione into cells by any other means.

Studies have shown that glutathione, taken by mouth, raises blood plasma levels of this antioxidant, which, by itself, has multiple health benefits. It also seems to be an established fact that glutathione from certain foods or supplements benefits our mitochondria—microscopical "organelles" inside cells, which generate the energy for many life processes.[5] But the jury is still out on the extent to which immune cells—lymphocytes, natural killer cells, and macrophages—can benefit from orally ingested glutathione.

Furthermore, orally taken glutathione "pro-drugs" or precursors like cysteine or NAC (N-acetyl-cysteine)—from which cells, theoretically, could also manufacture glutathione—are toxic. Our friends Durk Pearson and Sandy Shaw, authors of the famous pioneering book *Life Extension,* are of the opinion, though, that cysteine's toxicity can be avoided by simultaneously using other antioxidants to prevent its volatile sulfur from oxidizing.

Be that as it may, the proven ability of biologically active whey protein to provide glutathione to cells and tissue makes it a truly ideal delivery system. All the more so, since, at the same time, its immunoglobulins become available to our noncellular, or humoral, part of the immune system. In that case, their presence results in increased antibody production and, hence, in an all the more vigorous immune response.

Whey Protein Concentrate for AIDS and Central Nervous System Diseases

Certain conditions, notably AIDS, are intimately linked to depleted glutathione levels in T-cells and other defender cells of our immune system. It is therefore vital to find ways to deliver glutathione to these immune system cells.

So it is good news that a small pilot study with HIV-seropositiv men showed that biologically active whey protein concentrate—and no other protein source, including soy, spirulina, and casein—was able to dramatically increase the glutathione content of their immune system cells and increase body weight. The researchers also commented on a "marked improvement" in the "subjective feeling of well-being" of these patients.

Other conditions associated with depleted glutathione levels are certain central nervous system diseases like Alzheimer's and Parkinson's, as well as multiple sclerosis. In all these cases, biologically active whey protein concentrate—but only undegraded and, hence, biologically active whey protein—should be seriously considered as a promising, adjunct nutritional therapy since there is at present virtually no medical treatment for these conditions.

Biologically Active Whey Protein's Anticancer Effects

During the 1980s, several test tube studies, as well as animal experiments, showed an antitumor effect of whey protein concentrates. In line with these earlier studies, a 1995 Australian rat study comparing the effect of different diets on artificially induced tumors showed that "[undenatured] whey-fed animals had the highest concentrations of glutathione in their immune system cells and tissue and the most tumor protection."[6]

More dramatically yet, two Canadian researchers (Baruchel and Viau, 1996) have pointed out in a test tube study with rat breast cancer cells that biologically active whey protein concentrate is able to selectively deplete tumor cells of glutathione, while sparing normal tissue."[7]

To more fully appreciate all this, one has to keep in mind that glutathione levels in tumor cells are well known to be much higher than in normal cells. It is as if tumor cells have an uncanny sense of glutathione's ability to detoxify harmful substances, such as those used in chemotherapy, to destroy cancer cells. At any rate, for chemo- or radiation therapy to be effective, a certain drug is often first used to deplete cancer cells of gluthathione. The trouble, however, is that this drug depletes not only cancer cells of glutathione, but healthy, normal cells as well.

What makes biologically active (undenatured) whey protein concentrate (or isolate) so special is that—in and by itself, without need for anything else—it depletes only cancer cells of glutathione, but not normal tissue cells.

It is now also known by what mechanism this fortuitous effect is achieved. As the researchers point out, "glutathione synthesis in cells is inhibited by its own synthesis." Since glutathione levels in cancer cells are much higher than in normal cells, it is easier for their glutathione to reach the level where the negative feedback mechanism kicks in and no further glutathione is absorbed. When tumors are thus deprived of glutathione, their growth is inhibited and patients do better.

Best of all, this beneficial effect can be achieved simply by ingesting 10 grams of biologically active (undenatured) whey protein concentrate (or isolate), without having to use any harsh drugs with their inevitable side effects.

Actually, this fortunate effect of biologically active whey protein had already been noticed in another, slightly earlier Canadian study with cancer patients, although the mechanism by which it was achieved still escaped the researchers.[8]

In that clinical study, seven patients with various types of cancer (breast, pancreatic, and metastatic liver cancer) were, for six months, given 30 grams a day of powdered, biologically active whey protein. However, because of the relatively large amount of whey protein used (10 grams is the normal dosage), these patients were—to avoid kidney damage—put on an otherwise low-protein diet. This precaution was especially important because protein-overload can also encourage tumor growth.

Interestingly enough, it turned out that the two patients with the highest initial glutathione blood levels experienced the greatest improvement in terms of quality of life and performance. In fact, all the patients experienced an "[initial] period of improved sense of well-being." But with those patients whose glutathione levels in blood lymphocytes—and hence, presumably, also in tumor tissue—started to rise again, the cancer progressed as well.

These findings indicate again that biologically active whey protein selectively depletes cancer cells of glutathione. For that reason alone—if we may be excused for stressing the point—whey protein recommends itself as a nutritional adjunct to chemotherapy or radiation therapy. This applies particularly if any of the platin-type drugs are used, because they have a truly devastating effect on glutathione levels in healthy tissue.

The Bottom Line on Whey Protein

From the review of scientific literature, it is no exaggeration to state that whey protein concentrate or isolate is unrivaled as a high-protein source for human nutrition. Even leaving aside, for now, its immunity-enhancing potential if consumed in its biologically active (undenatured) form, whey protein is in a class by itself, even if it is not biologically active.

Just consider its many wellness-promoting properties: building of lean muscle mass, weight control (up or down, depending on whether used with a low-calorie or high-calorie diet), cholesterol-lowering effect, antiatherosclerotic function, bone growth, and improvement of bone strength. These are health benefits no other single food can claim.

If one now adds biologically active whey protein's

immunity-enhancing and anticancer properties to all that, it is no longer just an ordinary food but qualifies as one of the new "designer foods" or "nutriceuticals" you may have heard about—a kind of cross between a food and a drug. As such, biologically active whey protein has, again, no equal in terms of versatility, multiple health benefits, and even cost-effectiveness ($2.00–$3.00 a day, at current prices).

So, what to do?

Frankly, if you are—like us, at this time—just interested in whey protein only for what it does aside from boosting immunity, it is perfectly okay to use "regular" (largely denatured and, hence, not biologically active) whey protein concentrate or isolate. Eberhard, for instance, uses it mainly as an adjunct to the antiosteoporosis drug Fosamax. Aside from that, we also use it as about the best nonmeat protein source, aside from tofu (bean curd), in our semivegetarian diet.*

If you want to use whey protein in its guaranteed biologically active form, though—for instance, to fight HIV infection, cancer, Parkinson's or Alzheimer's disease, or MS—we know of only one source for such a product: Immunocal (from Immunotec Research Ltd. (1-800-786-1771; or www.immunocal.com).

How to Use Whey Protein Concentrate

Whey protein concentrates or isolates, in the usual quantities (approximately 10 grams, or 1 heaping tablespoon per serving), can be dissolved in water or any other nonalcoholic beverage. But do NOT use a blender; the mechanical agitation can denature the whey protein. So, even if you use regular—in all likelihood already largely denatured—whey protein, it is still a good idea not to use a blender, for it would degrade it even further.

You can also mix your whey protein into cold or luke-

*Health food stores carry various brands of powdered whey protein.

warm cooked cereal, as we do. It also blends well into nonfat or low-fat yogurt, while improving its taste and texture.

For additional health benefits—especially intestinal health—it is also a good idea to add a small amount (¼ teaspoon per serving) of FOS (fructo-oligosaccharides) to your whey protein drink, cereal, or yogurt mix (see Chapter 40).

NOTES

1. Takada, Y., et al. *Biochemical Research Communications,* June 14, 1996; 223 (2):445–49.
2. Zhang, X., and A. C. Beynen. Lowering effect of dietary milk–whey protein vs. casein on plasma and liver cholesterol concentrations in rats. *Brit. J. Nutr.,* 1993; 70:139–46.
3. Kajikawa, M., et al. Lactoferrin inhibits cholesterol accumulation in macrophages mediated by acetylated or oxidized low-density lipoproteins. *Biochem. Biophys. Acta,* 1994; 1213(1): 82–90.
4. Bousnous, G., and Ph. Gold. The biological activity of undenatured dietary whey proteins: role of glutathione. *Clin. Invest. Med.,* 1991; 14: 296–309.
5. Bousnous, G., S. Baruchel, J. Falutz, and Ph. Gold. *Clin. Invest. Med.,* 1993; 16:204–209.
6. McIntosh, G. H., et al. Dairy proteins protect against dimethylhydrazine-induced intestinal cancers in rats. *J. Nutr.,* 125:809–816.
7. Baruchel, S., and G. Viau. *In vitro* selective modulation of cellular glutathione by a humanized native milk protein isolate in normal cells and rat mammary carcinoma model. *Anticancer Research,* 1996; 16: 1095-11.
8. Kennedy, R. S., G. P. Konok, et al. The use of a whey protein concentrate in the treatment of patients with metastatic carcinoma: a phase I–II clinical study. *Anticancer Research,* 1995; 15:2643–50.

Chapter 41

Green Tea: Best Drink in the House

In the spring of 1991, experts from around the world gathered for two days in New York for an international symposium on the health effects of green tea.* They agreed that green tea offers a long list of health benefits, from helping to prevent tooth decay, lowering blood pressure, and lowering cholesterol levels to providing cancer protection, stabilizing blood sugar, and blocking the action of many carcinogens.

Admittedly, some of the claims about the alleged anticancer effect of green tea are based on studies with cancer cells that have been cultured in test tubes, or on studies with laboratory animals, rather than on clinical experience with tumors in real

*The symposium was sponsored by the American Health Foundation, an independent nonprofit research organization. So we can be quite sure of the general absence of bias in the findings of the participants.

people. Some, though, are based on comparing cancer and other disease rates among populations that consume a lot of green tea, such as the Chinese and Japanese, with those in populations, like ours, where green tea is not commonly drunk. The Japanese, who are avid green tea drinkers, have much lower death rates from all cancers than people in coffee-drinking countries. In fact, drinking green tea has helped reduce the exceptionally high rate of stomach cancer in Japan, which is largely due to their diet high in grilled foods* and salt.

But why is green tea rather than black tea credited with this medicinal effect? Well, both types of tea are made from leaves of the same plant (*Camellia sinensis*), but green tea undergoes less processing than black tea, thus preserving more of the beneficial plant compounds, called polyphenols. Green tea therefore contains 300 to 400 mg of these biologically active polyphenols (the most important being epigallocatechin) compared with 150 to 200 mg per cup of black tea. In other words, black tea is good for you, but green tea is better.

Unfortunately, the custom of adding milk or cream and plenty of sugar to black tea results in a health deficit rather than a health credit. On the other hand, strong black tea is so bitter—because of the tannins in it—that it is difficult to enjoy drinking it "straight." So, let it be skim milk or low-fat milk, and use a minimum of sweetener—preferably honey, if the choice is between honey and refined sugar. Among artificial sweeteners, choose aspartame-containing Equal, over saccharine-containing Sweet'n Low. (There is a warning on Sweet'n Low packages, printed in the smallest of small prints, in red on a pink background, making it almost impossible to decipher, even with a magnifying glass, which reads: "Use of this product may be hazardous to your health. This product contains saccharine, which has been determined to cause cancer in laboratory animals.")

*The high heat in grilling and frying turns proteins into carcinogenic compounds (pyrolisates) that attack the delicate mucous lining of the stomach. Continued exposure of this kind can lead to stomach cancer, as is often the case in Japan.

Also, green tea contains about a third less caffeine than black tea. But don't worry too much about the caffeine, even in black tea: researchers at the tea symposium said that the amount of caffeine in either type of tea was of minimal health consequence to most consumers. Even black tea contains only about half the caffeine in coffee, and most regular tea drinkers soon get used to the slight temporary increase in blood pressure that may occur—but usually doesn't. In fact, only a small percentage of people with high blood pressure may be adversely affected by it.[1] (For them it may be better to use decaffeinated green tea extract, which confers the same health benefits.)* In the long run, though, for most people, green tea has a blood pressure–lowering effect.

One of the most interesting participants in the green tea symposium was Dr. Junshi Chen of the Chinese Academy of Preventive Medicine in Beijing. He said that both Fujian oolong and jasmine teas inhibited the development of esophageal cancer. (Oolong and jasmine are somewhere between black and green tea, in terms of processing and content of active polyphenols; jasmine, flavored with jasmine blossoms, is a specialty tea made mostly with green or oolong tea.) Dr. Junshi Chen also explained that there are more than one hundred varieties of tea in China, the most widely used ones being (unfermented) green teas, jasmine tea, fermented black teas, and semifermented oolong.[2]

As for health benefits, Dr. Chen points out that all of the teas are clearly dose-dependent—the more tea—especially green tea—you drink, the greater the protective effect, particularly against cancer. That, at least, is what rat studies and population comparisons have shown.

Although the mechanism by which green tea protects against cancer is not fully understood, Dr. Chen lists the following points about it:

*The Life Extension Foundation offers such a green tea extract (1-800-544-4440), as does NAC Vitamin Co. (1-888-622-8532). Health food stores also offer different brands of green tea extracts.

1. It inhibits the binding of certain carcinogens to the DNA of the affected tissue (for instance, the liver, the lung, or the stomach).
2. It enables certain enzyme systems to stop the "promotion" process of cancer, preventing development from the first or "initiation" stage to the second or "promotion" stage. Green tea boosts the body's glutathione S-transferase system, which acts to detoxify cancer-promoting chemicals, and also seems to increase the enzyme activity of superoxide dismutase (SOD), resulting in better protection against DNA-damaging free radicals.
3. It also increases the level of PMN cells, a type of white blood cells that scavenge free radicals.

Several American studies confirm these Chinese findings. A group of researchers at the Skin Diseases Research Center at the University Hospitals of Cleveland, found that skin tumors artificially induced in mice by various cancer-causing chemicals, as well as ultraviolet radiation, were prevented by the addition of epigallocatechin (the active ingredient in green tea) to the drinking water of mice. They also cite several other studies that obtained positive results in a variety of laboratory animals against induced lung, forestomach, colon, duodenum and esophageal cancers simply by substituting green tea for the usual drinking water.[3]

Still other scientists, connected with the Medical College of Ohio and the University of Toledo, have more recently (1997) discovered yet another important anticancer mechanism of green tea: "Human cancers," they say, "need proteolytic [protein-"digesting"] enzymes to invade cells and form metastases. One of these enzymes is urokinase (uPA). Inhibition of uPA can decrease tumor size or even cause complete remission of cancers in mice." They then point out that EGCG (epigallocatechin-gallate), as in green tea, while being a weaker uPA inhibitor than some pharmaceutical uPA inhibitors, is, by contrast, nontoxic. In addition, its relative weakness can be compensated for by the consumption of greater amounts of green tea. They conclude that "the well-known anticancer activity of green tea is driven by inhibition of uPA, one of the most frequently overexpressed [overactive] enzymes in human cancer."[4]

Aside from the anticancer effects of green tea, a Japanese study with dogs confirmed that green tea protects against tooth decay and gingivitis by working like an antibiotic against several strains of bacteria known for causing these common dental problems.[5] The scientists cite other Japanese researchers who examined the effects of oolong tea extract in humans. They confirmed the antimicrobial effect of the extract and concluded that five major polyphenol compounds (including epigallocatechin) in green tea "may be useful in the prevention of oral diseases."

According to Lester A. Mitscher, Ph.D., of the University of Kansas,[6] green tea's numerous, well-documented health-protective merits include the following:

1. It contains epigallocatechin-gallate (ECGC), one of nature's most powerful polyphenol antioxidants.
2. It not only lowers levels of (bad) LDL cholesterol but also prevents its oxidation, which is a greater risk factor than the LDL cholesterol level itself.
3. It can have an overall blood pressure–lowering effect, inhibit blood clotting, and significantly reduce a person's risk of heart disease and stroke—but only if several cups are drunk daily!
4. It enhances immunity by activating several immune system components, such as B cells, T cells, and NK (natural killer) cells.
5. It has a powerful anticancer effect.

The message of all this is loud and clear: Switch from coffee to tea, especially green tea, and the jasmine and oolong varieties. Moderate coffee drinking may not do much harm—but tea will actually do you good, and be at least equally good tasting.

If all of that does not make green tea the best drink in the house—what would?

NOTES

1. Brody, Jane E. *The New York Times*, 14 March 1991.
2. Chen, Junshi. The antimutagenic and anticarcinogenic effects of tea, garlic and other natural foods in China: a review. *Biomed. & Environmental Scis*, 1992; 5: 9–12.
3. Katiyar, S. K., R. Agarwal, and H. Mukhtar. Protective effects of green tea polyphenols administered by oral intubation against chemical carcinogen-induced forestomach and pulmonary neoplasia in A/J mice. *Cancer Letters*, 1993; 73: 167–72.
4. Jankun, J., St. H. Selman, and S. J. Swiercz. Why drinking green tea could prevent cancer. *Nature,* vol. 387, June 5, 1997; 561.
5. Isogai, E., H. Isogai, et al. Effect of Japanese green tea extract on canine periodontal diseases. *Microbial Ecology in Health & Disease,* vol. 8, 1995; 57–61.
6. Mitscher, L. A. *Health,* vol. 12, no. 6, June 1998.

Chapter 42

The Sugar That's a Fiber That's Really a Sugar

If you have never heard of the tongue-twisting scientific term "fructo-oligosaccharides," don't worry. Most people—even the most health-conscious among us—haven't heard about it, either. But we are sure you will hear a lot about it in the near future.

If we were living in Japan, rather than in America or Europe, we would have all known about fructo-oligosaccharides long ago. "Neosugar," as it's called there, has been a household word in that country for years. Japanese scientists were the first to develop this special "sugar," and it is now used there in 450 different food products, from soft drinks and candies to cookies, puddings, cereals, chewing gum, and pancake syrup to infant formula. It's a $5 billion-a-year business and catching on fast here, too.[1]

But what does "neosugar"—or fructo-oligosaccharides, or

FOS—really consist of? Where does it come from? Is it a natural substance or man-made?

Oligosaccharides are natural types of carbohydrates present in a large number of fruits, vegetables, and grains. They can, for instance, be extracted from bananas, tomatoes, garlic, onions, Jerusalem artichokes, barley, and soybeans. If called fructo-oligosaccharides (FOS), it simply means they are made from fruits.

So, why not just eat the fruits and vegetables that contain these wonderful substances, rather than taking supplements that are made from them? The answer is that it would take thirteen bananas, eleven onions, or sixteen tomatoes to get the same benefits as provided by one teaspoon of FOS.

The more important question is what do the Japanese know about fructo-oligosaccharides (FOS) that we don't. In other words, why use FOS at all?

The answer is that many diseases originate in the gastrointestinal (GI) tract. All too many people on the typical high-fat/low-fiber American or Central European diet suffer from an unhealthy intestinal microflora, resulting in an overgrowth of putrefactant bacteria and "leaky gut syndrome." That, in turn, allows disease-causing bacteria and fungi to get through the intestinal mucous barrier and into the bloodstream, where they can cause any number of medical problems.

As is to be expected, an unhealthy intestinal microflora can lead to intestinal disorders such as irritable bowel syndrome, spastic colon, and mucous colitis. Worse yet, "bad" (pathogenic) bacteria produce putrefactive fermentation in the colon, which, in turn, results in the formation of liver toxins like ammonia and carcinogens like nitrosamines and secondary bile acids. FOS helps prevent these diseases in the intestine.[2]

An unhealthy intestinal environment can even upset our psychological well-being and cause mood disorders like depression, irritability, and hyperaggressivity. The reason, as researchers recently discovered, is that we have a "second brain" in our gut. That lower "other" brain can upset the larger upper brain as much as the upper brain can upset the lower brain, giving us "butterflies in the stomach," diarrhea, cramps, or constipation.[3]

A sick and unhappy gut—overgrown by "bad," putrefactant bacteria—is now also suspected of being a contributing factor in such autoimmune diseases as arthritis and rheumatoid arthritis, chronic fatigue syndrome, lupus, multiple sclerosis, fibromyalgia, and even diabetes mellitus. What FOS can do, however, is help the good *bifidobacteria* and lactobacteria to keep the bad bacteria in check and prevent or limit their attachment to the gut mucosa, thus helping to maintain a healthy intestinal environment.[4]

The best way to keep a healthy intestinal environment is to use FOS in conjunction with *lactobacillus sporogenes* (instead of or in addition to yogurt). This probiotic organism produces lactic acid, the body's natural germ fighter, and is more effective than acidophilus. Our source for it is America's Finest (1-800-350-3305).

NOTES

1. Bornet, R. J. Undigestible sugars in food products. *Am. J. Clin. Nutr.*, 1994; 59 (suppl.) : 7635–95.
2. Hidaka, H., et al. Effects of fructo-oligosaccharides on intestinal flora and human health. *Bifidobacteria Microflora,* 1986; 5:37–50.

   Hidaka, H., and T. Eida. Roles of fructo-oligosaccharides for the improvement of intestinal flora and suppression of production of putrid substances. *Shokuhin-Kogyo Food Eng.*, 1988; 31: 52.
3. Blakeslee, S. Complex and hidden brain in the gut makes cramps, butterflies and valium. *The New York Times*, 23 June 1996, Science section.
4. Alles, M. S., et al. Fate of fructo-oligosaccharides in the human intestine. *Brit. J. Nutr.* 1996; 76: 211–21.

Chapter 43

Mushrooms: Giving or Fighting Cancer?

With mushrooms there is good news and bad news. First the bad news: We discovered, to our dismay, that most mushrooms contain poisonous, carcinogenic compounds called hydrazines. They are developed by the mushrooms to defend themselves against being eaten by animals.

First the bad news: In a telephone interview with Dr. Bela Toth, a biologist at the University of Nebraska and the country's foremost expert on hydrazines, he told us of a Swedish colleague who analyzed no fewer than forty-eight edible European mushroom varieties and found that two-thirds of them contained these dangerous compounds.

Most of these powerful toxins are, fortunately, destroyed by cooking—undoubtedly the reason why we get away with eating them at all. The disturbing part about it, however, is that in America people use the white button champignon cut raw into salads, or as hors d'oeuvres, either stuffed or with a dip, not realizing the cancer risk they are taking!

One type of hydrazine, though, called agaritine, present in some of the most commonly eaten mushrooms, is destroyed only halfway by cooking. So even by eating only cooked mushrooms, we are still at some risk.

The trouble is that agaritine is converted in the body into a highly reactive, mutagenic metabolite that is able to produce stomach tumors in mice at disturbingly low doses, as Dr. Toth explained to us. We therefore get very upset when seeing people blissfuly eat raw mushrooms, thus getting a double dose of carcinogens, without an inkling that they are endangering their health.

Now the good news: While there are carcinogenic compounds in the majority of mushrooms, some mushrooms have anticancer, antiviral, antifungal, and blood pressure-lowering properties. Unfortunately, none of them are native to the Americas and Europe, but only to Asia, notably China and Japan. Moreover, most of them come more under the heading of "alternative medicine" than food. Nonetheless, we shall discuss some of the most important ones here, since they are, strictly speaking, not "nutritional supplements," either.

Shiitake

The Japanese shiitake mushroom (*Lentinus edodus*) has everything going for it: It tastes great, is highly nutritious, and has powerful anticancer and antiinfectious properties.

As for nutritional value, shiitake has twice the protein and soluble fiber of any other mushroom, three times the mineral content, especially calcium, phosphorus and iron, and plenty of B-vitamins and vitamin D-2.

Shiitake is the best-known medicinal mushroom in America and Europe because, unlike all the others (except for the black tree fungus, *mo-ehr* or *mu-er*), shiitake mushrooms are used primarily as a gourmet food, much appreciated for their delicate flavor, and only secondarily for their medicinal properties.

But shiitake happens to be—along with the rei-shi and maitake mushrooms—one of the most promising "alternative" and "adjunct" cancer therapies. At least two groups of researchers from Japanese universities, including scientists from the Mushroom Research Institute of Japan, have studied the shiitake mushroom. What they found is that extracts from shiitake suppressed tumor cell proliferation in liver tissue of experimental rats and "significantly raised the survival rate" of rats with liver cancer.[1]

The primary therapeutic compound in shiitake, just as in "seaweeds," appears to be a complex sugar (polysaccharide), in this case one called *lentinan*. This compound has been shown to boost interleukin-1 and interferon production (interleukin-1 and interferon are released by white cells of the immune system when fighting off virus attacks) which may, to a large extent, be why it has been found to act as a powerful immune system stimulant.

Medical researchers from the Metropolitan Institute of Medical Sciences, in Tokyo, and from Teikyo University, in Kawasaki, recently made the following exciting discoveries: "Lentinan . . . from *Lentinus edodes (Berk.) Sing.* [shiitake], an edible mushroom, has a marked antitumor activity . . . [it] suppresses chemical and viral tumorigenesis [tumor development] and prevents cancer recurrence or metastasis after surgery in animal models . . ."[2]

The same report goes on to summarize the effects of lentinan therapy with human cancer: "Results of the clinical application of lentinan [in humans] have proved prolongation of life span of the patients with advanced and recurrent stomach cancer and breast cancer. Lentinan also showed an excellent therapeutic effect in patients with advanced esophageal and squamous cell lung carcinoma in combination with surgery and irradiation. Lentinan protects patients from the side effects of radiotherapy and improved various kinds of immunological parameters with no toxic side effects in animal models and humans."

The most fascinating thing about all of this is how lentinan produces these remarkable, curative effects. In standard medical chemotherapy, toxic chemicals are supposed to kill the cancer cells. Before being approved, they are first tried *in vitro* (in the test tube) and if they kill cancer cells or inhibit tumor growth there, they are tried in animals, and finally in humans.

With lentinan and most other natural remedies, exactly the opposite is the case. As in the case of lentinan, they frequently do not work *in vitro* at all, but only *in vivo,* that is, in the live organism. The Japanese researchers therefore concluded, "Lentinan has no direct cytotoxic [cell-killing] effect against target cells [cancer cells] and its effects are host-mediated." In other words, the benefit comes from the interaction of the therapeutic substance (say, lentinan) with the organism's own immune defenses.

The active ingredient in shiitake mushrooms, lentinan, apparently gives our immune system such a powerful boost that it results in preventing the development of cancer and metastases, as well as shrinking the tumors themselves. Nobody seems to know exactly how this works; we only know that it does work.

Other studies have shown that lentinan's ability to protect against radiation can be put to great advantage in radiation therapy to shield patients from the notorious and often very damaging side effects of this type of treatment. Similarly, if lentinan—and certain other medicinal mushroom extracts—are used as adjuncts to chemotherapy and radiation, they can significantly increase a patient's survival time.

In the case of chemotherapy, Japanese scientists have a pretty good idea why this is so: they think that certain natural compounds in lentinan (and apparently in other medicinal mushroom extracts as well) react with the chemotherapy drugs, producing a synergystic effect by creating other powerful cancer-fighting compounds.[3]

Lentinan, unfortunately, is not available in America and Europe. In contrast, in Japan, lentinan (produced by the huge

Japanese chemical company Ajinomoto) is officially approved by the health authorities for the treatment of stomach cancer. (In actual medical practice, it is also used in combination with chemotherapy and radiation for other types of cancer.)

Fortunately, a number of concentrated shiitake products are available here on the health food market, as is the shiitake mushroom itself—especially in its dried form. All of these can be quite effective if used correctly. So, cancer patients can benefit from shiitake by using it on their own either to protect themselves from the side effects of radiation or to increase the effectiveness of chemotherapy. Others may use shiitake, in one form or another, to protect health in other ways—to lower cholesterol or blood pressure, for example.

Shiitake has also been found to have strong antiviral activity,[4] which should make it a candidate for adjunct therapy in virus-related cancers, such as certain leukemias, papilloma virus–related cervical and rectal cancers, and even HIV. In addition, an antifungal compound[5] has recently been isolated from shiitake, making shiitake therapy all the more promising in mixed infections.

Best of all, there is ample evidence from several Japanese animal studies that not only the purified extract, lentinan, but also the mushroom itself is effective in fighting cancer when added to the feed of mice.[6] Again, it is not too far-fetched, in this case, to extrapolate from these animal studies to the human situation, because the physiology of mice is, in this respect, not too different from our own.[7]

How to Use Shiitake and Other Medicinal Mushrooms

One of the best ways of using shiitake mushrooms (or, for that matter, any medicinal mushrooms) is—according to time-honored Chinese medical tradition—to prepare a concentrated broth from them. Dried mushrooms (available from many health food stores and Asian food markets), rather than fresh ones, are preferable for that purpose, because the dried mushrooms provide, ounce for ounce, more of the mushroom's active ingredient(s)—either lentinan or other, as-yet-unidentified compounds.

The trick is to first either grind up or cut up the dried mushrooms as finely as possible. Only then do you simmer them slowly in good, unchlorinated water, until you think the broth has become sufficiently concentrated. (To prevent digestive stomach acids from interfering with the compounds in shiitake or other medicinal mushrooms, we suggest drinking the broth between meals, rather than with other food.)

Another way of getting most of the benefits of pure, chemically extracted lentinan (the pure shiitake essence) is to take freeze-dried shiitake concentrate in capsule form. There are several such products on the health food market. The trouble is that some of them contain a lot of dextrose (corn starch) as a carrier for the actual shiitake granules. So you have to read the labels carefully.*

Aside from that, the tasty, fresh shiitake mushrooms can be enjoyed sauteed in olive oil or canola oil, or with your green salads, in soups, with scrambled egg whites, and in a number of other ways. The only trouble is that your average American or European food market is not likely to offer fresh shiitake (though more and more of them do). But dried shiitake mushrooms from health food stores or Chinese groceries are quite acceptable if soaked overnight in unchlorinated water to soften them before cooking.

*We favor a product called "Shiitake Plus" from Carotec, Inc. (P.O. Box 9919, Naples, FL 1-800-522-4279), which is an encapsulated form of pure, freeze-dried shiitake mycelium. Chinese herbal stores also offer concentrated shiitake powder in capsule form, but it is harder to assess its purity and concentration. A Chinese herbalist would be your best guide to the right product.

The Tree Fungus Mo-ehr

We had already called attention to the heart-protective effects of the Chinese black tree fungus mo-ehr (or mu-er) in the first edition of *Formula for Life* and have been using it for years in soups and salads. Then, in 1991, *The New England Journal of Medicine* published a paper about the mo-ehr's just discovered anticlotting effect, suggesting that it may be helpful in fighting heart disease.[8]

The New York Times reported on all this in a front-page article and immediately the price of a bag of dried fungus, the way it is sold in New York's Chinatown, doubled overnight. Subsequently, it was found that this tree fungus also protects against cancer.[9] (The Chinese merchants seemed to have missed that news, so the dried mo-ehr is still quite affordable, even after the big 1991 price increase.)*

The Japanese Rei-shi/Chinese Ling-zhi Mushroom

As Dr. Ralph Moss writes in his earlier cited book, *Cancer Therapy,* scientists discovered that the rei-shi (or ling-zhi, pronounced ling-je) mushroom contains a unique protein, called ling-zhi-8 (LZ 8), after the Chinese name of the mushroom. A water-extract, or concentrated broth, of rei-shi has been found to inhibit tumor growth in animals.[10]

We had a curious personal experience involving the rei-shi (or ling-zhi) mushroom we would like to share with you. It concerns a woman friend of ours with a history of breast cancer,

*The dried tree fungus mo-ehr (also called mu-er), imported from China, is sold in many Chinese markets. In New York's Chinatown it is, for instance, offered at Wah Yin Hong Enterprises, 232 Canal St., New York, N.Y. 10013. Phone: 212-941-8954 (between $3 and $4 for a six-ounce bag).

who was, at the time, in postoperative chemotherapy at Memorial Sloan-Kettering Cancer Center, in New York.

Initially, like the vast majority of cancer patients, she was totally uninformed about adjunct cancer treatments. More recently, however, (thanks to our "subversive" influence), she became quite knowledgeable about adjunct treatment options that could be used in conjunction with chemotherapy and radiation.

As it happened, her oncologist at the cancer center was Chinese but thoroughly Westernized. So one day, after a chemotherapy session, she suddenly popped the "loaded" question, "Tell me, doctor, how do you think a Chinese physician would treat me if I were in China?"

He almost panicked. Then he said in a low, almost whispering voice, as if the walls in this citadel of orthodox cancer therapy might have ears, "Well . . . in China you would probably be given some herbal medicines, along with chemotherapy."

"Oh," she said, "what kind of herbal medicines?"

"Well," he said, "they have all kinds of them."

"But what traditional medicine do they use most, in a case like mine?" our friend kept pressing him.

At first, the doctor seemed at a loss how to reply. Finally he said, "What I think they mostly use with cancer are certain mushrooms." However, he didn't know what any of these mushrooms were called.

On the way home from the clinic, however, our friend happened, by sheer coincidence, to pass by a Chinese herb store. The recent conversation with her Chinese-American oncologist still very much on her mind, she impulsively went in and naively asked the elderly Chinese man behind the counter whether he had any Chinese mushrooms that were good for cancer.

The man was very reluctant to answer her, she said. He undoubtedly knew full well that if he offered this American lady—for all he knew she might be an FDA decoy, trying to entrap him—anything supposedly "good for cancer," he could lose his business and might even go to jail.

It was only after she told him frankly that she was a cancer patient, and related her conversation with the Chinese-American doctor to him, that the man, who turned out to be the store owner, started to relax. Still, he took the precaution of saying he had no "cancer medicine," but having said so, opened one of the cupboards and took out a wooden box containing dried mushrooms.

"Some of my Chinese customers who have cancer are making a tea from this mushroom," he said.

"What is the name of it?" she asked.

He mentioned a name that sounded to her like "linje," she said. Of course, it turned out to be none other than ling-zhi (the Chinese name for the Japanese rei-shi mushroom).

Our friend was too confused to buy the mushrooms, and that's where our story ends. But we found that most Chinese medicine stores sell dried ling-zhi (*Ganoderma lucidum*).

We once bought a box of a dozen of these dried mushrooms, put six of them in water to soak overnight, and naively thought of using them next day, cut into scrambled egg whites, the way we are using the shiitake. To our surprise, however, these mushrooms didn't want to soften up much, even after soaking all night. So we decided to consume them, the traditional Chinese way, by boiling them for about half an hour, and just drinking the broth.

That gave us our second surprise: the broth was bitter as gall! That's how we found out that ling-zhi (rei-shi), though classified as edible, is really more medicine than food.

Maitake

The Japanese mushroom maitake (*Grifola frondosa*)—the latest arrival on the mushroom front—is now also available here on the health food market.

It is said to be an even more powerful cancer fighter than shiitake and rei-shi (ling-zhi). The truth, however, is that while the large, basketball-sized maitake mushroom has, for centuries, ranked high in traditional Japanese folk medicine, there exist, as yet, not nearly as many scientific studies on it as on shiitake and rei-shi (ling-zhi).

Nonetheless, there is some preliminary scientific evidence that maitake is indeed effective against some cancers and thus a good condidate for adjunct (supportive) therapy. Moreover, it appears that maitake is active not only when its extract is administered by injection, or administered orally,[11] but also when eaten as the mushroom itself (said to be rather good tasting).[12] But all of these promising results have yet to be confirmed by further studies before we can be more certain.

Still another problem is that maitake, which is ultrascarce in nature, has been commercially raised, in Japan, only a short time, so supply is still limited and prices quite high. But anyone interested in preventive medicine should closely follow the research on this mushroom.

Other Medicinal Mushrooms

Actually, there are at least a dozen other Japanese and Chinese mushrooms, for which research has shown similar cancer-inhibiting effects, as in the case of shiitake, rei-shi, and maitake. Most of them are, however, as yet used only experimentally by doctors in Japan and China, and are not available in the West at all. They are, therefore, of little practical importance to us now, although some of them appear to be powerful immune system boosters and cancer-fighters.

There is, however, one mushroom, or rather fungus—*Coriolus versicolor*—which does have practical implications for us Westerners, even now. A polysaccharide powder from this fungus is marketed in Japan under the brand name Krestin or PSK, as an anticancer drug.* Where allowed (in the United States it is, of course, *not* allowed), it is frequently combined in cancer therapy with chemotherapy drugs like mitomycin-C, carbaquone, and others.

*Krestin is produced by Kureha Chemical Industry Co., Ltd., Tokyo.

A number of studies have shown that, when so used, it improves the effectiveness of chemotherapy, for instance, in leukemia and post-surgical treatment of colorectal and stomach cancers.[13]

NOTES

1. Takehara, M., et al. Isolation and antiviral activities of the double-stranded RNA from Lentinus edodes (Shiitake). *Kobe J. Med. Sci.*, 1984; 30: 34–35.

   Sugano, N., et al. Anticarcinogenic actions of water-soluble and alcohol-insoluble fractions from culture medium of Lentinus edodes mycelia. *Cancer Lett.*, 1982; 17: 109–14.
2. Maeda, Y. Y., H. Yonekawa, and G. Chihara. Application of lentinan as cytokine inducer and host defense potentiator in immunotherapy of infectious diseases. In *Immunotherapy of Infection*. New Delhi, India: National Institute of Immunology: 261.
3. Obeidi, F., et al. Synthesis and actions of a melanotropin conjugate, Ac-[Nle4, Glu(gamma-4'-hydroxyanilide)5, D-Phe7]alpha-MSH4-10-NH2 on melancytes and melanoma cells in vitro. *J. Pharm. Sci.*, 1990; 79: 500–504.
4. Takehara, M., et al. Antiviral activity of virus-like particles from Lentinus edodes (Shiitake). Brief report. *Arch. Virol.*, 1979; 59: 269–74.

   Takehara, M., et al. Isolation and antiviral activities of the double-stranded RNA from Lentinus edodes (Shiitake). *Kobe J. Med. Sci.*, 1984; 30: 25–34.
5. Takazawa, H., et al. An antifungal compound from "Shiitake" (Lentinus edodes). *Yakugaku Zusshi,* 1982; 102: 489–91.
6. Chihara, G., Y. Y. Maeda, J. Hamuro, T. Sasaki, and F. Fukuoka. Inhibition of mouse sarcoma 180 by polysaccharides from *Lentinus edodes*. *Nature,* 1969; 222: 637–38.

   Nanba, H., and H. Kuroda. Antitumor mechanisms of orally administered shiitake fruit bodies. *Chem. Pharm. Bull.,* (Tokyo), 1987; 35: 2459–64.

   Nanba, H., et al. Antitumor action of shiitake (Lentinus edodes) fruit bodies orally administered to mice. *Chem. Farm. Bull.* (Tokyo), 1987; 35: 2453–58.
7. Nanba, H., and H. Kuroda, op. cit.

   Takehara, M., et al. Antitumor effect of virus-like particles from Lentinus edodes (shiitake) on Ehrlich ascites carcinoma in mice. *Arch. Virol.,* 1981; 68: 297–301.

   Nanba, H., et al., op. cit.

8. George, J., and S. Shattil. The clinical importance of acquired abnormalities of platelet function. *NEJM,* 1991; 324: 27.
9. Moss, Ralph W. *Cancer Therapy*. NY: Equinox Press, 1992; 278.
10. Maruyama, H., et al. Antitumor activity of Sarcodon aspratus (Berk.) S. Ito and Ganoderma lucidium (Fr.). *Karst. J. Pharmacobiodyn.,* 1989; 12: 118–23.
11. Ohno, N., et al. Two different confirmations of antitumor beta-glucans obtained from Grifola frondosa. *Chem. Pharm. Bull.,* Tokyo, 1986; 34: 2555–60.

    Hishida, I., et al. Antitumor activity exhibited by orally aministered extract from fruit body of Grifola frondosa (maitake). *Chem. Pharm. Bull.,* Tokyo, 1988; 36:1819–27.

    Nanba, H. Antitumor activity of orally administered "D-fraction" from Maitake mushroom (Grifola frondosa). *J. Naturopathic Med.,* 1993; (4) 1:10–15.
12. Ibid.
13. Oh-hashi, F., et al. Effect of combined use of anticancer drugs with a polysaccharide preparation, Krestin, on mouse leukemia P388. *Gann.,* 1978; 69: 255–57.

    Tsugagoshi, S., et al. Krestin (PSK). *Cancer Treatment Rev.,* 1984; 11: 131–55.

    Fujii, T., et al. Treatment with Krestin combines with mitomycin C, and effect on immune response. *Oncology,* 1989; 46: 49–53.

    Nakazata, H., et al. Clinical results of a randomized controlled trial on the effect of adjuvent immunotherapy using Esquinon and Krestin in patients with curatively resected gastric cancer. Cooperative Study Group of Cancer Immunochemotherapy, Tokai Gastrointestinal Oncology Group. *Gan To Kagaku Ryoho,* 1986; 13: 308–18; 14: 2758–66.

    Hasegawa, J., et al. Inhibition of mitomycin c-induced sister-chromatid exchanges in mouse bone marrow cells by the immunopotentiators Krestin and Lentinan. *Mutat. Res.,* 1989; 226: 9–12.

    Nakazata, H., et al. An effect of adjuvant immunochemotherapy using Krestin and 5-FU on gastric cancer patients with radical surgery (first report)—a randomized controlled trial by the cooperative study group. Study Group of Immuno-chemotherapy with PSK for Gastric Cancer. *Gan To Kagaku Ryoho,* 1989; 16: 2563–76.

Part Seven

"Unfriendly" Foods

In the preceding chapters, we have been considering some important but little-known facts concerning health-protective and immunity-boosting foods. But it is not enough to eat more of the "right" kind of foods; we also have to know what "wrong" foods to avoid. That's why, in the chapters that follow, we shall give you the vital facts about what makes these "no-no" foods so dangerous to our health.

Chapter 44

Barbecued, Grilled, and Fried Foods

The worst of these three cancer-causing cooking methods is barbecuing. Unfortunately, it is also one of America's obsessions—as is the equally problematic grilling of meats over an open fire, for instance, to make kebabs, an import from the Near East that has spread like wildfire in both America and Europe.

We love life too much to eat these kinds of high-risk foods. For one thing, they have been exposed to too much high heat. That produces chemical burn products of proteins that are known carcinogens. As scientific research has shown, an average, half-pound, well-done steak, broiled over charcoal, contains as much cancer-causing benzopyrene as 150 cigarettes![1]

As the fat drips down onto the red-hot charcoal or wood during barbecuing or grilling over fire, a cloud of smoke goes up and literally coats the meat on the grill with a layer of highly carcinogenic chemicals (polycyclic aromatic hydrocarbons). Some people might say, So what? But it has been shown that the risk for pancreatic cancer (one of the worst) increases in proportion to the frequency with which fried or grilled meats are eaten.[2]

We still remember with a mixture of horror and amusement how hard it was for us, on a book tour in the deep South, to find food in the hotels and restaurants that wasn't barbecued, grilled, or deep fried. The trouble with deep-frying is that the breading around the food becomes literally saturated with fat. Secondly, by subjecting the oil to such high heat, the fatty acids are broken down and oxidized. This produces dangerous oxygen radicals in these molecularly altered fats. If we now eat foods that have been fried in this way, together with the fat-saturated breading, we are not only getting far too much fat, but are also exposing ourselves to the cell-destructive activity of free radicals.

Are we therefore to abstain from all deep-fried foods? Not necessarily. One can remove the breading and eat only the inside parts that have not been as directly exposed to the hot fats, as the outside crust has. This is our strategy, for instance, when served deep-fried fish or chicken.

Our own preferred cooking methods, however, are steaming, boiling, broiling, and baking. On the other hand, we are no "purists" and do not like to create problems when eating out. Nor is there really any need for doing so, since there are feasible compromises, like the example we just gave, that do not seriously affect our health.

NOTES

1. Zapsalis, C., and R. A. Beck. *Food Chemistry and Nutritional Biochemistry*. NY: John Wiley & Sons, 1985: 1061.
2. Norell, S. E., A. Ahlholm, R. Erwald, et al. Diet and pancreatic cancer: a case control study. *Am. J. Epid.* 1986; 124: 914–15.

Chapter 45

FATS DO MORE THAN MAKE YOU FAT

For decades, the medical establishment resisted the constantly accumulating findings—not only from outsiders like Nathan Pritikin but also from within medical ranks—that there was a direct correlation between fat consumption, especially of saturated animal fat, and degenerative diseases like atherosclerosis, coronary heart disease, diabetes mellitus, and cancer.

Today, all of that is of course no longer a matter of serious dispute. Ironically, though, general acceptance of the fact that saturated fat is "bad" for us has led to a change in many people's eating habits that has exposed them to even greater health risks.

Many people (the authors included) switched from using saturated fats, like butter and lard, to unsaturated vegetable oils and margarine. They thought themselves safe in doing so. In actual fact, though, they jumped from the frying pan into the fire! True, unsaturated vegetable oils cannot clog up our arteries with cholesterol, because they don't have any. But they are much more prone to oxidation and hence the production of cancer-causing free radicals.

Free radicals are known to attack the DNA in the nucleus of cells, thus causing cellular abnormalities (mutations)—the precondition for cancer. So, the depressing net result of substituting such polyunsaturated (highly unsaturated) vegetable oils like the popular safflower, corn, sunflower, or cottonseed types of oil for saturated animal fats is that we are reducing the chance of developing atherosclerosis and heart disease by increasing cancer risk. Not much of a bargain, if you ask us.

What to do? The message is simple but does not seem to be getting through to any but the most health-conscious among us: use only virgin olive oil or canola oil for cooking and salad dressings.

They, too, are unsaturated, like the other vegetable oils. The difference is, they are not "polyunsaturated" but only "monounsaturated," which means they are much less prone to oxidation than their polyunsaturated cousins. That's why olive oil and canola oil are the only vegetable oils that are heart-protective, while not exposing you to more cancer risk.

Margarine—made from hydrogenated vegetable oils—is really no safer than butter with regard to heart disease. The vegetable fats lose their unsaturated molecular structure during the hydrogenation process, giving them their harder, butter-like consistency. Unfortunately, however, hydrogenation produces trans-fatty acids, which our bodies are not used to. Recently, scientists at Harvard University have shown that these trans-fatty acids are a major factor in heart attack and stroke.

Butter, on the other hand, not only has cholesterol, but also increases triglycerides, another type of fatty acid, in the blood stream. Furthermore, a 1993 Japanese study has shown that eating butter interferes with the body's ability to dissolve blood clots, as well as affecting blood platelet function.*

We stopped using butter and margarine long ago and don't miss either one. However, by the time you read this, there should be a new and entirely different kind of margarine available that not only has no cholesterol, but can actually lower your cholesterol! We are referring to Bennecol, a Finnish invention, using modified plant sterols.

There are at least five major clinical studies, published in prestigious scientific journals such as the *Journal of Lipid Research, Clinical Science,* and *The New England Journal of Medicine,* all supporting the producer's claim that a daily intake of 25 grams of this margarine "significantly lowers serum total and (the "bad") LDL cholesterol blood levels without altering (the "good") HDL, when consumed as part of a healthy diet."[1]

While we are on the topic of fat substitutes, a quick word about Olestra. It is mostly used to replace the vegetable oils that are normally used in producing potato chips and tortilla chips. Although it is FDA-approved, we remain skeptical. Olestra, writes Marian Burros in *The New York Times,* "travels through the body scooping up the fat-soluble vitamins A, D, E and K, as well as nutrients like carotenoids [such as beta-carotene and lycopene], which are found in fruits and vegetables and which some people believe help prevent cancer."

Sure, Procter & Gamble, producers of Olestra, are putting some of the depleted vitamins and nutrients back in. But as one critical scientist put it, "We do not know which substances to replace, how much to replace, the bioavailability of replacements or the biological activity of newly described carotenoids."†

To say it once again, all saturated animal fats, but especially

*Kozima, Y., et al. Impaired fibrinolytic activity induced by ingestion of butter: Effect of increased plasma lipids on the fibrinolytic activity. *Thrombosis Research*, 1993; 70: 191–202.

†Dr. Sheldon Margen, Professor Emeritus of Public Health Nutrition at the University of California, San Diego, as quoted in *The New York Times,* 25 Jan. 1996.

the fats in red meats, are highly problematic. "Marbled" steak, so favored by steak fanciers, with whitish veins of fat running through it, is obviously the type highest in fat. If the meat has been "hung" or "aged" (supposedly to "improve" its taste), its fats are thoroughly peroxidized and loaded with free radicals, ready to turn our normal, healthy cells into abnormal, premalignant ones. Such altered cells only need another little push from one cancer-promoting factor or another—say, an environmental pollutant—to turn into full-blown cancer.

But even free radicals are not the whole reason why cancer likes animal fats, present in meat, luncheon meats, whole milk, full-fat cheese, butter, and so on. These fats also increase the number of certain strains of anaerobic bacteria in the gut that produce toxic, carcinogenic substances.

> "The more beef and animal fat you eat, the greater is the potential for the production of more carcinogens in the colon."
>
> —Charles B. Simone, M.D., M.S.S., oncologist

The only relatively safe meat, sorry to say, is that from wild animals that have not been deliberately fattened, and are therefore much leaner than cattle. As much as we regret the killing of any animals, it has to be said, in all fairness, that as long as the consumption of domesticated cattle is allowed, there is no reason to forbid the sale of meat from game animals, as America does. In fact, a case can be made for the necessity to periodically "cull" certain wild animal populations, like deer, which might otherwise run out of feed, or do too much damage to crops.

The Trouble with Hamburger

We cannot leave this discussion without telling you why America's (and now the world's) beloved hamburger has to be at the top of any health-conscious person's no-no list:

- hamburger meat is very high in saturated fat and cholesterol
- grinding the meat exposes more surface to the air, encouraging oxidation and the generation of free radicals
- the grinding breaks up the red blood cells in the meat, releasing iron and copper ions that catalyze the production of still more cancer-initiating free radicals
- the high heat involved in frying or grilling the ground meat turns its protein molecules into carcinogenic chemicals[2]
- if the ground meat has been exposed not only to high heat, as in frying, but also to smoke, as by grilling or barbecuing, it adds a cloud of highly carcinogenic hydrocarbons to this already high-risk kind of food

The reason we are so "paranoid" about fat is, as the quotation from Dr. Charles Simone on the preceding page points out, that it has been convincingly linked in many scientific studies to ovarian, prostate, and colon cancers.* These findings keep being confirmed and reconfirmed. Just recently, for instance, researchers at Memorial Sloan-Kettering Cancer Center in New York City found that human prostate cancer tumors grew only half as fast in mice with diets of about 21% fat as in mice with diets of about 40% fat, which is the level of fat consumed by many Americans and Europeans.

The moral of all this? Well, if the idea is to prevent or survive cancer, atherosclerosis, diabetes mellitus, and all the

*In 1982, for instance, the Committee on Diet, Nutrition, and Cancer of the U.S. National Research Council declared that high-fat diet involves increased risk of breast, colon, and prostate cancers.

other nutritional and lifestyle diseases, one had better stay away from such suicide foods as hamburgers, marbled steaks, fatty sausages, and all the rest.

Most cakes, cookies, and full-fat ice creams are also loaded not only with hidden fat, but also sugar. Surely, there are other, less lethal pleasures in life. But tradition, habit, denial, and commercial interests conspire in favor of these high-risk foods.

NOTES

1. *Food Processing,* Feb. 1997; 53–54.
2. Sugimura, T., M. Nagao, T. Kawachi, et al. Mutagen-carcinogens in food, with special reference to highly mutagenic pyrolytic products in broiled foods. In *Origins of Human Cancer,* H. H. Hiatt, J. D. Watson, and Winsten, eds. Cold Spring Harbor, NY: Cold Spring Harbor Laboratory, 1977; 562.

Chapter 46

Red Meat: Is It Worth the Risk?

In the preceding chapter we discussed the health hazards posed by the high fat content of meats. Here we only want to remind the reader that not only marbled steak, roast beef, ribs, and similar high-fat meats are definite "no-nos" on a health-protective diet, but also popular luncheon meats such as corned beef, pastrami, bologna, and all the rest. (It is tempting to be cynical and say foods like that qualify for a warning from the Surgeon General: "This Food May Be Dangerous to Your Health.")

The devil of it is that fats carry the flavors, so the fatter the meat, the "better" it tastes and the greater its popularity. But, in this chapter, we will talk not about the dangers of the fat and cholsterol in meat, but about another, totally independent and only very recently discovered danger to our health from red meat.

Unfortunately, that applies even to the leanest of lean red meat. In other words, you can buy the leanest cuts on the market, trim off all the remaining fat, and the problem remains!

What is it about red meat (apart from its saturated fat) that is so bad for us?

Fact 1: Scientists have known for some time that the amount of iron (serum ferritin) stored in our bodies has something to do with the risk for coronary heart disease and heart attack (myocardial infarct).

Fact 2: In 1992, a Finnish study demonstrated a link between dietary iron intake and serum ferritin concentration (one of the main forms in which the body stores iron), with acute myocardial infarction (heart attack).[1]

Fact 3: In 1994 came the publication of a large-scale study of male health professionals, which found a connection between the consumption of food containing a certain type of iron, called heme iron, that is present only in meat—especially red meat—and heart disease and stroke.[2] (Vegetables, fruits, cereal grains, seeds, nuts, and dairy and soy products, as well as eggs, only have another benign form of iron, called non-heme; chicken has only about 40% of heme iron, and fish none.) In other words, red meat is the primary source of "bad" heme iron in the diet, and this factor is independently linked to cardiovascular disease.

Fact 4: Unfortunately, the heme iron is well absorbed by the body and any excess stored in tissue. This accumulation is now known to be the basic cause of red meat's effect on heart disease and cancer, quite aside from the effects of the fat in meat.

In contrast, the "good," non-heme iron, ironically, is under strict regulation by the body's control system. If you take in more non-heme iron than you need, the body simply stops absorbing it and excretes it. So most people get plenty of the "bad" iron from red meat, which is readily absorbed and stored in the body, while getting much less of the "good" iron from vegetarian sources.[3]

Fact 5: Red meat is rich in the amino acid methionine, from which the body produces another amino acid called homocysteine, which builds up in the blood.[4] This compound has now been found to be about the worst thing to have at high levels in the body, because it is a powerful factor in the hardening of arteries (atherosclerosis) and the buildup of arterial plaque, as well as hypertension—all high-risk factors for heart disease, heart attack, and stroke.[5]

Women (more precisely, premenopausal women) have a certain (though by no means total) degree of protection in these respects because their monthly loss of blood reduces the buildup of homocysteine in the bloodstream.[6] The same has been found with men who regularly donate blood. (An instance in which altruism has concrete health benefits!)

Fact 6: Men and women who consume red meat daily have a 60% greater chance of dying from coronary heart disease than those who consume red meat less than once a week.[7] In contrast, the results of several additional studies have shown that vegetarians run far less risk of developing heart disease.[8] When beef was added to a vegetarian diet, the result was increased blood cholesterol, especially of the "bad" LDL kind that produces arterial plaque, and a rise in systolic blood pressure.[9]

Fact 7: Some people (perhaps as many as 12%) have a genetic defect that produces an inefficient form of an enzyme that normally breaks down at least some of the homocysteine and renders it harmless. But if you eat red meat and happen to be one of the 12% or so who have this genetic defect, you would be in double jeopardy of heart attack and stroke.

The good news is that certain B-vitamins, specifically folic acid and vitamin B-6 can also break down the dangerous homocysteine. In fact, when Dr. Rima Rozen, a geneticist at McGill University in Montreal, who had been involved in the genetic studies that led to this discovery, found out that she was one of the 12%, she couldn't get to the health food store fast enough to buy some folic acid and vitamin B-6.

Fact 8: Red meat consumption has also been found to be associated with prostate cancer. One study found that men who consumed red meat at least four times a week had almost double the mortality rate from prostate cancer as a matched group of vegetarian men.[10]

A similar link was found between red meat consumption and breast cancer, colon cancer, kidney cancer, stomach cancer, and pancreatic cancer. But this is undoubtedly a result not only of high homocysteine levels but of the high fat content of meat, which has long been known to promote cancer.[11]

Fact 9: The good news is that homocysteine concentrations in the body can, as we have seen, easily be corrected by taking folic acid and vitamin B-6 supplements, as provided on our nutritional supplement program.

The other good news is that there is no need to eat red meat, since there are so many good-tasting alternatives for protein, especially for semi-vegetarians like us, who allow for some seafood, poultry, and low-fat dairy products—not to forget the richest protein source of all—whey protein concentrate.

NOTES

1. Salonen, J. T., et al. High stored iron levels are associated with excess risk of myocardial infarction: eastern Finnish men. *Circulation,* 1992; 86: 803–11.
2. Ibid.
3. Kushi, L. H., et al. Health implications of Mediterranean diets in light of contemporary knowledge. 2. Meat, wine, fats, and oils. *Am. J. Clin. Nutr.,* 1995; (suppl.): 1416S–27S.
4. Kushi, L. H., ibid., 1417S.
5. Brody, Jane E. Folic acid emerges as a nutritional star. *The New York Times,* 1 March 1994. Science section.
6. Sullivan, J. L. Iron and the sex difference in heart disease risk. *Lancet,* 1981; 1:1293–94.

7. Snowdon, D. A., et al. Meat consumption and fatal ischemic heart disease. *Preventive Med.,* 1984; 13:490–500.
8. Cheng, C. J., et al. Mortality pattern of German vegetarians after 11 years of follow-up. *Epidemiology,* 1992; 3: 395–401.
9. Sacks, F. M., et al. Effects of ingestion of meat on plasma cholesterol of vegetarians. *JAMA,* 1981; 246:640–41.
10. Phillips, R. I., et al. Association of meat and coffee use with cancers of the large bowel, breast, and prostate among Seventh-day Adventists: preliminary results. *Cancer Res.,* 1983; 43(S):2403–2408.
11. Kushi, L. H., et al., op. cit. 1417S–19S.

Chapter 47

What to Do About Salt

There was a time when we, like many other people, thought that salt is bad only for people with high blood pressure. Wrong! The vital fact is that salt—beyond a certain minimum that is quickly reached because everything we eat contains some salt—is harmful to everybody. Especially, though, to cancer patients, HIV-positives, and older people.

There has been lots of medical controversy about whether salt is really the main culprit in producing high blood pressure. Obviously, one's genetic makeup and lifestyle, as well as the amount of stress a person's physiology has to handle, all have to do with hypertension (high blood pressure). But recent studies with chimpanzees in Africa have shown indisputably that adding salt to the animals' diet sent their blood pressure through the ceiling. When salt was removed, blood pressure came back down.*

Dr. Derek Denton of the University of Melbourne, Australia, reported in the October 1996 issue of *Nature Medicine* that we humans evolved to handle up to approximately 3 or 4 grams of salt a day, but no more. Most people in the United States and Europe, though, consume between 10 and 15 grams of salt a day, most of it from commercially processed foods. That is far too much. But Dr. Denton warns against cutting back on salt too abruptly, which could have serious side effects.

It is scary to think that there are populations who consume even more salt than Americans and Europeans. People in some rural Japanese communities, for instance, consume about 26 grams a day. A shocking 39% of these people over age forty suffer from high blood pressure, and death from cerebral hemorrhage is common.

Our concern, however, is not only with the hypertensive effects of salt, but with its other "unfriendly" qualities as well.

Salt's Effect on Life Span

There is no longer any doubt that salt shortens life. Experiments have shown that rats on a high-salt diet had a median life span several months shorter than those given less salt. Translated into human terms, this difference represents a shocking thirty-two-year shortening of our life span—even without the presence of cancer, or any other special risk factors.

Salt and Osteoporosis

Another fact that is not sufficiently understood is the link between salt intake and osteoporosis. As is well known, osteopo-

*Study of Chimps Strongly Backs Salt's Link to High Blood Pressure. *The New York Times,* 3 Oct. 1995.

rosis is the major underlying cause of bone fractures, affecting especially postmenopausal women and older people in general. About 1.5 million osteoporosis-related fractures occur in the United States a year, many of them resulting in disability and even death. Yet, there is little public awareness of the connection between these sad statistics and salt consumption.

There is now evidence that osteoporosis prevention has to start with reduction of salt intake during a person's youth. One study, carried out in young girls between eight and thirteen years of age, for instance, clearly showed that high salt intake reduces calcium retention in bones and is a predictor of future osteoporosis.[1]

A two-year longitudinal study with postmenopausal women, likewise, left no doubt that bone loss by these women could be "significantly reduced by halving their sodium intake." The study also showed that this preventive effect on bone loss can be even more dramatic by simultaneously cutting down on salt and doubling calcium intake (for instance, by taking calcium/vitamin D-3 supplements).[2] Needless to say, regular, weight-bearing exercise (brisk walking, low impact aerobics, etc.) is still another important preventive factor.

The Trouble with Processed Foods

Unfortunately, many people are too busy to regularly prepare their own food and are therefore dependent on processed foods, such as "TV dinners" and similar frozen or canned foods, which all have high salt content. The trouble is that food manufacturers, fearing customer rejection, are very resistant to reducing the salt content of their products. You therefore have to carefully read labels and select processed foods with the lowest sodium content, for instance, the Pritikin or "Weight Watchers" line of prepared foods.

It's true, some of these foods are awfully bland if eaten as is. But one can always add a little soy sauce, Bragg Liquid Aminos, and spices to make them more palatable.

Using More Potassium Makes Salt Less Dangerous

Another fact that is not sufficiently appreciated is the important sodium/potassium balance of our bodies. The problem is that when we raise our sodium intake by eating too much salt (sodium chloride), we simultaneously deplete the potassium level in our cells. This heightens the risk from salt, because potassium neutralizes some of the toxic effects of excess sodium intake. Fortunately, it is easy to avoid a sodium/potassium imbalance simply by taking potassium supplements.*

Is Salt Addictive?

It doesn't take a genius to figure out why most of us eat too much salt. For one thing, salt has a habituating effect that comes close to addiction (as is, incidentally, also true for fats and sweets). We noticed how dependent we had become on salt only when we seriously started cutting down on it.

Secondly, when one eats a lot of salt, one does not notice when foods are oversalted. Studies have shown that there is absolutely no correlation between the amount of salt people think they are consuming and the amount they actually consume. (It is similar to people's perceptions of how much alcohol they drink!) We cannot, therefore, rely solely on our own judgment.

On the other hand, when you don't eat much salt, you immediately notice when there is more salt in the food than you are used to, like when eating out, or when you have accidentally

*A reasonable dose is 99 mg of potassium per day, for instance, as in Twinlab's potassium citrate and aspertate. Another way of supplementing potassium is by using a combination mail order product of 100 mg of magnesium, plus 99 mg of potassium (aspartate) by Vitamin Research Products.

oversalted a dish. This is not only the common observation of people on low-salt diets, but has been amply confirmed by scientific experiments.[3]

Being used to salty foods, most of us don't even notice that there is a lot of hidden salt in many of the foods we don't think of as particularly "salty," such as bread, most commercial salad dressings, and cheeses (even of the "light" variety).

Ways to Keep Salt Out and Taste In

Some people use some kind of "light" salt, which is simply a mixture of table salt (sodium chloride) and potassium. There is nothing wrong with this, if you don't mind the slight "off" taste of these mixtures (we do).

We much prefer seasoning our food, as earlier mentioned, with either low-sodium soy sauce, or Bragg Liquid Aminos (available in health food stores). These products also contain salt, but one tends to use much less of them because of their other strong flavors. For the same reason, using more spices, like rosemary, thyme, oregano, fenugreek, turmeric, curry, and so on, also reduces the need for salt.

As a substitute for high-fat and high-salt grated Parmesan cheese for flavoring pasta dishes, we sometimes use Sapsago cheese, a low-salt but delicious hard cheese, made in Switzerland from only skim milk, spices, and herbs as a substitute. It comes in three-inch-high cones, so you have to grate it yourself. Unfortunately—while popular in Europe—it is available in America only from the more sophisticated urban food stores and some health food stores.

Now that the media has brought to public attention how protective even commercial tomato sauce is with regard to prostate cancer, this is really the best way to eat our pasta dishes—provided we choose a low-sodium brand, or prepare it ourselves from fresh or sun-dried tomatoes, with only a minimum of salt or no salt at all.

NOTES

1. Matcovic, V., et al. Urinary calcium, sodium, and bone mass of young females. *Am. J. Clin. Nutr.,* 1995; 62:417–25.
2. Devine, A., et al. A longitudinal study of the effect of sodium and calcium intakes on regional bone density in postmenopausal women. *Am. J. Clin. Nutr.* 1995; 62: 740–45.
3. *Toxicants Occurring Naturally in Foods*, 2nd ed. Washington, D.C.: National Research Council, National Academy of Sciences, 1973; 31–32.

Chapter 48

WHAT TO DO ABOUT SUGAR

As with salt, one obviously also has to watch one's intake of sugar. But, personally, we are much less worried about sugar than we are about salt. Sugar is, after all, the only kind of food that the brain can use. Nor have we ever seen a scientific study showing—contrary to the case with salt—that sugar, per se, shortens the life span of either laboratory animals or humans.

Nonetheless, sugar can be a problem, a big problem. Many American and European kids become little sugar addicts just as soon as they get off the breast or bottle. It therefore shouldn't come as a surprise that so many school age children are already suffering from diabetes mellitus, and often without either the parents or the school being aware of it.

Sugar addicted kids turn into sugar addicted grown-ups. With advancing age, that can lead to diabetes, contribute (via very-low-density lipoprotein production) to abnormally high cholesterol levels, and even aggravate existing cancer.

Cancer Loves Sugar

It is another vital but generally overlooked fact that cancer cells gobble up sugar much more greedily than normal cells do. In the normal digestive process, enzymes in our mouth, stomach, pancreas, and intestines slowly break down (metabolize) the complex sugars from grains, legumes, and vegetables into simpler and more easily absorbed sugars, like fructose, sucrose, and glucose (the end product of sugar metabolism).

Normally, as soon as there is a rise in blood glucose concentration, a negative feedback mechanism comes into play: insulin is secreted into the blood and any excess glucose is converted to glycogen and stored in the liver and muscles for use as needed. Other glucose is converted to fat and stored as adipose tissue.

Cancer cells, however, short-circuit this normal process by forcing the liver to produce more and more glucose for them from stored glycogen and the breakdown of fat and muscle cells. The end result of all this is the well-known abnormal glucose tolerance and increased glucose production in people with cancer, with the breakdown of fat and muscle resulting in the terrible wasting syndrome. (This is the exact opposite of what happens when healthy people experience weight loss due to food deprivation, as in fasting or starvation, where there is a *decrease* in total glucose production.)[1]

There is also some evidence that sugar may inhibit immune function. Studies indicate that sugar in the bloodstream can diminish the ability of phagocytic white cells to engulf and gobble up bacteria, viruses, and possibly cancer cells.[2]

It is for all these reasons that we try to avoid refined white table sugar as much as possible—not so much because of the sugar itself, but because the refining process involves the use of potentially mutagenic chemicals.

Practical Solutions

Instead of refined sugar, we now prefer honey, rather than Equal, which we had previously thought to be the answer to our sugar problem. Unfortunately, however, the sweetening ingredient in Equal (aspartame) contains the amino acid phenylalanine, which poses a certain risk for people (like Eberhard) who have or have had the skin cancer malignant melanoma, which happens to thrive on phenylalanine. (For others, however, the sweetener Equal seems to be perfectly all right.)

In our own case, though, honey seems to be a better solution, for only 30% of it is sucrose, the rest being about 40% fructose and 31% glucose ("sugar" is, of course, 100% sucrose). Admittedly, fructose and glucose are sugars too, but they are much more easily metabolized than sucrose and do not cause as strong a "hypoglycemic rebound" as table sugar.

Honey has also been successfully used in folk medicine for various ills, for example, to relieve bacteria-caused infant diarrhea. It might therefore also be useful with cancer- and AIDS-related diarrhea.

Nor is it too surprising that honey might have medicinal properties. Bees do, after all, produce honey from the nectars of a large variety of flowers, many of which are known to be medicinal. It is undoubtedly due to the subtle effect of these flowering plants and trees the bees feed on—like red clover, linden blossom, buckwheat, sheep sorrell, and goldenseal—that honey has been successfully used in folk medicine to treat various ills.

Moreover, the different flavors of honey—some stronger than others, depending on the flowering plants and trees the bees have been feeding on—let one use less of it than one would in the case of flavorless sugar. (This is similar to substituting strongly flavored soy sauce or Bragg Liquid Aminos for plain salt.)

As for ourselves, we now use small amounts of pure, raw honey for our breakfast cereal and other dishes that need some additional sweetening. We have yet to give two macrobiotic sugar substitutes—barley malt and brown rice syrup—a try. They should be great for making low glycemic index desserts like custards and puddings.)

We do not think it is a good idea to use presweetened, cold breakfast cereals. Our own breakfast consists of cooked whole oatmeal with added other grains like quinoa, amaranth, barley, and millet, plus wheat bran, barley bran, oat bran, or rice bran for extra fiber. We also use small amounts of cooked raisins and/or prunes as sources of additional soluble fiber.

NOTES

1. Cheblowski, R. T., D. Heber, B. Richardson, and J. Block. Influence of hydrazine sulfate on abnormal carbohydrate metabolism in cancer patients with weight loss. *Cancer Research*, Feb. 1984; 44: 857–61.
2. Sanchez, A., et al. Role of sugars in human neutrophylic phagocytosis. *Am. J. Clin. Nutr.,* 1973; 26: 1180.

   Ringadorf, W., et al. Sucrose, neutrophil, phagocytosis and resistance to disease, *Dent. Surv.,* 1976; 52:46.

   Bernstein, J., et al. Depression of lymphocyte transformation following oral glucose ingestion. *Am. J. Clin. Nutr.*, 1977: 30:613.

Chapter 49

Our Dietary Philosophy

Our personal—for lack of a better term—"antiaging" diet is not a rigid system of dos and don'ts. Nor is it ideologically driven, such as religious "vegetarianism," or the principles of "balance" between "yin" and "yang" foods, or "food combining," which forbids the simultaneous consumption of proteins and starches.

Instead, our only criterion for inclusion or exclusion of any food into what we believe to be a health-protective diet is whether it makes, as far as we can tell, nutritional sense, seems scientifically justified, and is relatively nondamaging to the environment.

In practical terms, our protective diet is eclectic, taking from different diets (for instance, from macrobiotics) what seems to recommend itself to logic and is generally in accord with current knowledge about nutrition.

Most important, our diet is not a static system, but something that is constantly open to revision, to experimentation and new discoveries. We think it is basically sound and seems to serve us well. At the same time, we are constantly learning and keeping our minds open to new dietary ideas and the discovery of new good-tasting and yet health-protective foods.

One must also keep in mind that no diet, no matter how good, can ever be the only right one for everybody. We are all different, and our individual digestive metabolisms differ widely—not to mention the enormous differences between individual tastes and food preferences. This is a fact also acknowledged by macrobiotics, which attempts to customize its basic diet to each individual's specific nutritional needs.

Especially in the case of serious illness, such as cancer and AIDS, people may have to adjust their diet (macrobiotic or otherwise) to maintain body weight and perhaps allow for somewhat more protein (for which whey protein concentrate would be ideal) and even for some fats than would normally be necessary or advisable. Still other people may need more fiber, or an adjustment up or down in the amount of raw foods. (It goes without saying that in all these special cases, one should seek professional guidance.)*

We therefore hope that sharing our basic diet, which is geared to the avoidance of the degenerative diseases of aging, will serve as general guidelines to more effective nutritional disease-prevention in general and cancer prevention and life extension in particular.

Obviously, proper nutrition must be the basis for any disease prevention or survival strategy. No alternative or conventional cancer or AIDS therapy, or even the best supplement program, can possibly succeed without being solidly anchored in sound nutrition.

*Since most doctors are, alas, not very knowledgeable about nutrition, and mainstream dietitians are trained within rather narrow parameters, our best advice to those looking for nutritional guidance is to get in touch with a macrobiotic center. Such centers can refer a person to a nutritional counselor, trained in the special requirements of people with serious illnesses.

To inform ourselves about nutrition and make the necessary adjustments in our customary ("conditioned") eating habits is therefore a mandatory first step toward disease prevention and life extension—no matter how many nutritional supplements we take and how much attention we pay to physical fitness through aerobics, working out at the gym, jogging, or whatever.

The final outcome of whatever else we may be doing to stay well and have a long and productive life, will, first of all, depend on what we don't eat, as on what we do eat. Second, it will depend on our total lifestyle. Third, it will depend on our mental/emotional state (absence of chronic anger, fear, anxiety, envy, and other negative emotions). Fourth, it depends on the quality of our human relationships, which is both a function of our emotional well-being, as well as its precondition.

Last but not least, we think our physical and emotional health depends on something for which our vocabulary fails us, but that can perhaps best be thought of as our spiritual well-being and the awareness of something infinitely greater than ourselves.

Part Eight

The Mind-Body Connection

Chapter 50

Mental Attitudes That Make the Difference

We have, in the first part of this book, focused exclusively on the physical things we can do to stay well and slow down the aging process. We have been talking about the right way to take vitamins and minerals, as well as what antioxidants, foods, and hormones can do for us. In short, we have considered just about everything on the physical plane to avoid disease and add the most years to our productive lives. Now it is time to look at the mental/emotional factors that can support all these wonderful physical life-extension strategies and make them work all the more effectively for us.

First, though, we should take a look at the flip side—the mental/emotional attitudes that can undermine our best efforts at staying well and enjoying a long and productive life. It is all the more important to do so, since we are often not fully aware of how we all can be, in these respects, our own worst enemies.

If positive, healthy mental attitudes are important for staying well, they are obviously even more important when we are ill, for illness puts a heavy stress on us. But regardless of whether we happen to be well or ill, it is not the stress itself—the stuff of life that comes our way—but how we react to it that makes the difference. We shall see, as we go on, how all this plays out in real life and how we can enlist our own minds to live to the limits of our personal, maximal life span.

We know a great deal today about how the way we think and feel about things affects, in ever so many ways, our neurological, endocrinological, and immune systems, which, in turn, affect how well or poorly every organ of our bodies functions, or fails to function. It has to do with how we digest our food, how we sleep, our blood pressure, how we cope with bacteria, viruses, and toxins from the environment, and all the rest. In short, our minds have a whole lot more to do with illness and wellness than we are normally aware of.

Let's take an example with which we are all familiar: chronic worry and anxiety, as everybody has had occasion to realize, can be very hard on our health. It makes us sleep poorly, upsets our digestive system, and makes us more susceptible to colds, the flu, and even to heart disease and cancer. More often than not, we can do precious little about the circumstances that make and keep us worried and anxious. In our society, with its "everybody for himself and the devil take the hindmost" mentality, there is chronic financial anxiety—how to make ends meet, job insecurity, unemployment, economic survival in old age, and the like.

Obviously, there is only so much—and it isn't very much—the individual can do about all this stress. It affects us all.

Other anxieties common in today's society—and not just ours—include parents' constant worries about their children's safety or whether they will be drawn into the drug culture. At the same time, children face worries about violence in the schools and how to deal with their emerging sexual urges in the face of peer pressure and the ever-present threat of AIDS.

In addition, parents must often cope with interpersonal

tensions, both at home and at work. There is so much marital discord and anger, and often it does not even end after protracted, bitter, and contentious divorce. And then there are the "children of divorce"—all too often the hapless victims of the parents' vicious custody fights—who have to cope with the stress of their divided loyalties.

One could go on and on about stresses that we can often do little or nothing about. We do have a certain measure of control, though, over our reactions to these circumstances. In other words, the stress is often an inescapable given. We cannot wish it away, or pray it away, or force it away. The only thing left is to try and modify our responses to the stress to minimize its impact on us.

Sometimes the stress to which we react with anxiety, fear, or anger is in the past and cannot hurt us anymore. But we react to it as if it were a very real and present danger and we could get hurt by it right here and now.

Eberhard, as the reader may recall, has had a couple of what he calls "close encounters with the big C." The first one—a diagnosis of multiple myeloma—fortunately turned out to be a false alarm. (He "only" had a precancerous colon tumor that was surgically removed, "just in time.")

The second one, a malignant melanoma on his hip, was for real. It had, of course, to be excised immediately, for melanoma is a very dangerous kind of skin cancer that can quickly metastasize. So he has to watch every little mole on his body, lest it be another melanoma lesion. That's perfectly normal; anybody who's ever had melanoma should always be vigilant and examine his body for any signs of recurrence. (Just as any woman who has ever had breast cancer should be all the more alert to any suspicious lumps or swollen lymph nodes.)

But it is easy to let one's fears get out of hand and become hypochondriacal at the least physical symptom. That, of course, produces more stress, which will produce more symptoms, which will lead to more anxiety and so on and so forth. In fact, this sort of vicious circle is able to produce a state of chronic anxiety and stress which, as we shall see, has profound effects on the immune system and can influence every aspect of our physical being.

The Physiology of Stress

We have seen how certain emotional states, like chronic anxiety, depression, and anger, as well as upsetting social circumstances—financial problems, unemployment, marital discord, divorce, geographical dislocation, bereavement—all produce stress. On the physical level, this results, among other things, in the release of corticosteroids (cortisol), which have a directly suppressive effect on the immune system.

More scientifically put, the "hypothalamic-pituitary-adrenal axis," which is responsible for regulating our hormonal secretions and neurological reactions, is highly sensitive to a variety of environmental and psychological stressors—just as the immune system is. Furthermore, all these physiological systems interact with one another, so that what affects one of them affects them all.

It is also well known that stressful emotions, like anxiety, anger, and fear, have a powerful effect on our lymphatic system, probably by way of neurotransmitters, which are hormone-like secretions that make connections between nerve endings. That, in turn, can affect many other physiological functions, including our entire sympathetic, as well as parasympathetic nervous systems.

For instance, fear can make our hearts beat faster, make us perspire, even have us temporarily lose urinary or bowel control. Anger, too, can have many effects on our bodily functions. There are many accounts of people having heart attacks while in a rage, and chronic anger can produce high blood pressure. Common expressions reflect these connections, as when we talk of rage making us "see red," or having "butterflies in the stomach," or when we say, "My heart jumped into my throat."

The reason for all of this is that emotional tension, anxiety, and anger produce increased sympathetic nervous system activity and increased levels of catecholamines (such as dopamine, epinephrine, and norepinephrine), all of which contribute to the classic "flight or fight" response. Now, if one lives in anxiety and fear, or in a chronic state of anger and suppressed rage, all one's physiological systems are constantly in the "red alert" mode—that is, they are under permanent stress.

Numerous animal studies have shown that even temporary stress can stop the immune system from functioning properly. In one experiment, blood samples from rats exposed to electric tail shock showed loss of lymphocytes (white cells of our immune system, produced by the thymus gland and bone marrow).

In another experiment, the rats were divided into three groups and all injected with a tumor-producing chemical. They were then exposed to either no electric shock, escapable shock, or inescapable shock. Predictably, the rats who received the inescapable shock were only half as able to reject development of a tumor and twice as likely to die of cancer as the rats in the other two groups.

Likewise, a number of experiments with university students showed that just taking final exams—by no means one of the most stressful situations in life—is already sufficient to impair lymphocyte function. Natural killer cells, in particular, which are thought to be our first line of defense against viral infections and possibly cancer, were "significantly suppressed." That is why so many students come down with colds and flu after exams.

With high levels of stress—whether it comes from the environment or our own emotions—there exists the potential for serious consequences, especially in those persons whose health is already impaired, as, for instance, in chronic illness or advanced age. It is therefore doubly important for anyone in that kind of situation to be especially mindful of the immunosuppressive effects of chronic anxiety and anger.

It is also worth mentioning in this connection that a habitually negative, pessimistic way of looking at things—really a form of depression—also keeps the immune system in a permanently weakened state. If one's aim is to protect one's health and enjoy a long and productive life, it is therefore important to consciously cultivate a positive, optimistic frame of mind and to decidedly reject negative modes of thought.

Can We Worry Ourselves Sick?

We recently came upon a fascinating article about Russian children who supposedly had been exposed to fallout from the Chernobyl nuclear reactor accident and were now treated in a Cuban clinic.[1] All of these children were sick all right, but the doctors there said that, with many of them, their physical problems had nothing to do with exposure to radiation—that most of them had not, in fact, been exposed—but were "clearly due to inadeqate nutrition and hygiene and from stress."

The children, however, uniformly attributed their medical problems to having been exposed to fallout. They suffered so much anxiety, though, that the doctors coined the term "radiophobia" for their condition. The children suffered from anxiety not only about their health, they said, but also about their future, even worrying whether they would ever be able to have normal children. "They live in a climate of fear," as one Cuban pediatrician put it; "if they get a headache, it's Chernobyl."

There is a curious American parallel to this. It concerns the psychosomatic effects of the much less dangerous nuclear reactor accident at Three Mile Island in 1979. Three years afterward, there was a "small wave of excess cancer" among people living in the vicinity of the plant. The increase in cancers, however, could not have been caused by radioactive fallout during the accident. This had already been established by a previous study.[2] The scientists at first speculated that this was caused by stress. And in fact, people living fairly close to the plant (less than four miles) reported feeling heightened stress in the months and years following the accident. But some scientists were skeptical that this stress could have triggered increased cancer growth directly. Instead, they suggested that it could have acted indirectly by sensitizing people toward symptoms and seeking medical care.

"In that case," they said, "the Three Mile Island accident could actually have done some people living close to the plant a favor by leading them to detect existing cancers sooner than they would have otherwise."[3]

That may well be so, but seems to underestimate the role of stress in disease. As Professor H. J. Eysenck, point out, "Of all the risk factors considered, stress and the individual's reaction to stress are showing the strongest correlation with death from cancer and CHD (coronary heart disease). "It is curious," he concludes, "that the medical profession has, on the whole, failed to pay much attention to the importance of stress and personality in the causation of disease and tends to reject claims that stress is a real killer."[4]

Is There a Stress-Prone Personality?

The reason why social scientists came to suspect the existence of a "stress-prone personality" was that some people continue to experience and report "stress," although others, in similar circumstances, do not. Take, for instance, a typical workplace situation: Company A has a number of employees who complain that they're "all stressed out": there's too much pressure, their supervisor is too demanding, working hours are too long, things are too hectic, one can't concentrate, there's too much noise, the office decor is depressing, the office furniture is uncomfortable, the lighting is bad, and so on.

Of course, the company could simply fire these unhappy, "stressed out" workers. That would be the easy solution. But these same workers often happen to be otherwise hard-working, conscientious, and reliable. So, in enlightened self-interest, the company decides to improve the work situation: working hours are made more flexible; lighter workloads are given those who claim they can't keep up with the work; people are given an option to be transferred to another department, if unhappy where they are; office walls are repainted in gay colors; more comfortable chairs are provided for employees spending many hours in front of computer terminals; lighting is improved, and green plants are put everywhere to cheer up the place.

Everybody happy? End of problem? Not by a long shot! Complaints continue, no matter what the company does to make things as pleasant as possible. That's when industrial and organizational psychologists and psychiatrists, like Dr. Thomas Pickering of Cornell University, and Dr. Osamu Fujita of Japan,[5] among others, started focusing on the workers themselves and not only on the work environment.

What these scientists found was that some persons are simply much more stress-prone than others. Moreover, they discovered that these people have five characteristics in common:

1. They tend to be rigid in their thinking, decision-making, and behavior; in short, they lack flexibility.
2. They are extremely achievement-oriented and find it hard to just relax and "do nothing." (They have no inner resources to meaningfully occupy their leisure time.)
3. They are overly anxious to please others and hypersensitive toward criticism.
4. They find it difficult to deal with frustration and aggression.

   Depending on the cultural context, they might tend to overreact, possibly yelling or even lashing out at other workers, as is the norm in America. Or they might turn the aggression inward and blame themselves if anything goes wrong, as is more common in Japan. In Germany, on the other hand, stress-prone workers are more likely to take their problems and frustrations out on themselves by developing psychosomatic illnesses, like nervous gastritis, colitis, asthma, eczema, and so on.
5. They tend to be unaware of their own problems and inclined to attribute their stress and distress solely to environmental factors. What these people need to understand is that it's not just outside factors that have to change—*they* may have to change, too.

So what has all this to do with illness, wellness, and longevity? Well, in the first place, the stress-prone personality is, by definition, also illness-prone. That is because of the effects of chronic internal stress on the immune system, as well as on the endocrinological and neurological systems—in short, on every aspect of human physiology.

Furthermore, the stress-prone personality is obviously not only more susceptible to illness, including cancer, but will be at a definite disadvantage in coping with serious illness. It is therefore of the utmost importance that anybody recognizing himself or herself as of this personality type get insight into their predisposition to overreact to stress and acquire better coping skills.

This is all the more important in today's world, in which outside (environmental) stress is perhaps worse than ever. A group of social scientists at Fordham University, for instance, have recently found that the U.S. "social health index"—that is, the degree of social ills in the country, like the gap between rich and poor, the number of uninsured, average weekly earnings, and the amount the elderly are paying for health care—are all at their worst levels ever.[6]

Avoidable and Unavoidable Stress

There is no doubt that wellness and longevity depend, to a large extent, on learning how to reduce one's own stress level. In fact, it is imperative for every one of us to see the urgency of a drastic change in our attitudes toward adversity. We absolutely have to learn to cope more effectively with perhaps unavoidable outside stress and to recognize and reduce self-created, and hence avoidable, internal stress.

We do not, for instance, have to nurture chronic anger, or compare ourselves with others who seem to be better off, and indulge in pointless envy, thus inviting Shakespeare's "green-eyed monster" into our hearts. Nor do we have to allow hostility to poison our minds and bodies, or contribute to interpersonal conflict. As the famous designer Eva Zeisel, now pushing ninety but as vibrant and creative as ever, said to an interviewer, "Eternity is only in the present, and when the present is filled with disharmony, it is lost."[7]

Most important, perhaps, we all have to learn not to stress ourselves out by useless worrying about things that are beyond our control. As Madame Jeanne Calment, who died at the ripe old age of 122, said, "If you can't do anything about it, don't worry about it." She was, as Jean-Marie Robine, a public health researcher who knew her well, said, "someone who, constitutionally and biologically speaking, was immune to stress."[8] Which reminds us of the religious philosopher J. Krishnamurti, who flatly stated, "I refuse to have any problems"—and meant it.

But, aside from obviously dysfunctional mental states, like chronic worrying and anxiety, anger, resentments, envy, and hostility, there are other kinds of destructive mental attitudes that are usually not suspected of being so bad. In fact, they are generally considered virtues rather than "vices." Take, for instance, such things as driving ambition and competitiveness, always having to be the first, the best, the most efficient one. Yes, such high-powered competitiveness may bring "success," power, and money. But it will inevitably take its toll on the overly ambitious person's mental and physical health, not to mention its fallout on marriage and family relations. So, perhaps it is better to be less ambitious (less "driven") and, hence, less "successful," and just live life more fully and enjoy the moment, even if it doesn't "get you anywhere."

Unfulfilled Goals and Survival

While ambition, if not balanced by other values, works against survival, going after an unfulfilled goal can be an important factor for longevity. It can even be a mechanism for survival in the case of life-threatening illness. The late British playwright Dennis Potter (*Pennies from Heaven, The Singing Detective,* etc.) comes to mind in this connection. While terminally ill with pancreatic cancer, he gave a last interview on BBC. He explained to the interviewer, Melvyn Bragg, a well-known British TV personality, that rushing to finish the two plays he was working on was the most important thing for him now. "My only regret would be," he said, "to die four pages too soon."[9] That goal kept him going till he had finished the plays.

Another example is the British conductor Jeffrey Tate, who is suffering from a congenital and painful spinal malformation that has left him partially crippled and causes his internal organs to be permanently compressed. While the condition is not life-threatening in an immediate sense, Mr. Tate is clearly aware that it is bound to shorten his life span considerably. The one thing he wanted to accomplish in life was to conduct Wagner's entire *Ring Cycle,* and he did.

"The awareness that I'll possibly have a short life span," he told an interviewer, "has acted on me both positively and negatively. The negative side is that ever since my childhood, I've had terrifying moments when I've suddenly felt acutely aware of the fact of death. The positive side is that I've tried to live as intensely as possible. I entered into my forties with great relish, sensing that I was coming into my own as a conductor. But now, as I enter my fifties, I feel that I have yet other goals . . . I can no longer put things off. There are books I will need to read, places I will need to visit, people I will want to see . . ."[10]

Of course, not all of us can have such lofty and "creative" goals as conducting Wagner or writing plays. But the nature of the unfulfilled goal or dream does not matter. It may be going after that college degree one always wanted to get but never had time for. Or the painting or pottery class one was interested in, but never got around to. Or the trip one had always wanted to take, but that only remained a fantasy, or whatever unrealized goals we may have. All such things can help us live more fully, or serve us to survive in the face of serious illness, while others, without such goals or uncompleted tasks, often lose all incentive to live and just allow themselves to deteriorate and wilt away.

To "Stay in the Running"

Another big mistake made by many people—especially older people or those of us who have to cope with serious illness or its aftermath—is to figure that they can no longer exercise to keep in better physical shape, because their bodies, weakened by illness, accident, or age, no longer tolerate any kind of exertion. That, of course, is often the painful reality. But frequently we give in too easily to physical incapacities, or it is more a matter of perceived rather than realistic incapacity.

Take, for instance, the long-distance running champion Mark Conover. At the height of his promising career he was diagnosed with Hodgkin's disease, a lymphatic cancer that had invaded his lungs and chest. He underwent chemotherapy for five months that made him lose all his hair. But he made a joke of it, pulling out clumps of hair in front of people and saying, "I've got to quit this job; there's too much stress!"

After chemotherapy he felt completely depleted, but soon started running again. "I just wanted to feel the wind blowing against my face, to feel alive, instead of staying on the couch and feeling miserable," he said. Gradually he increased his workouts to one hundred miles a week—an unbelievable distance for a recent cancer survivor! He admittedly now tires a lot more during the last few miles, but it was, he said, "a relief to run that well." It gave him a sense that life—normal life, that is—was far from over: he was still very much "in the running."

"What Mark did is applicable in everybody's life," said Jeff Berman, president of Cancer Support Services, an organization that encourages exercise as a way to cope with disease. "Most people diagnosed with cancer are afraid to lift a finger, thinking they will get a recurrence or worse. Mark is a prime example of empowering yourself, taking control and being as fit as you can possibly be in terms of helping to recover."

Guilt and Self-Blame

Often guilt and self-blame accompany illness or accidents. In the case of illness, we may blame ourselves for not having taken better care of ourselves, or indulging in "unfriendly" foods like fats and sweets, not exercising enough, not trying hard enough to kick the nicotine habit, drinking too much, maybe even taking hard drugs.

If we have been injured in an accident, we are apt to tell ourselves things like, "I should have never . . ."; "I ought to have known better . . ."; "I had no business to . . ."; and so on.

That may all be very true, but what good is this guilty hindsight going to do? Dwelling on the mistakes of the past and beating up on ourselves only lead to depression and internal, self-generated stress, which undoes nothing, is debilitating, and only makes things worse.

To be sure, we have all done foolish things in our lives, sometimes very foolish things. But the only thing that matters is how we conduct ourselves right now, in the present. If we have truly learned from our mistakes, we are not likely to repeat them. That does not mean we won't make other mistakes. Chances are, we will. But as long as we keep learning and come to understand better and better how it is that we are making certain mistakes, the less we will be tempted to repeat them. And that's what personal growth is ultimately all about.

Characteristics of the Adaptive Personality

The adaptive personality—in constrast to the stress-prone personality, who feels powerless, easily threatened, and overwhelmed—is resilient and not easily intimidated. She feels in control and does not doubt her ability to cope with adversity.

Adaptive people are not afraid or too rigid to make the necessary adjustments that changed circumstances—for instance, geographic dislocation, loss of one's job, breakup of a relationship, protracted illness—may dictate. People like this are always ready to reinvent themselves when the need arises.

Most important, the adaptive personality does not rail against unfortunate situations or indulge in self-pity (the "Why me?" mentality). Instead, they use whatever happens—no matter how upsetting, difficult, and unpleasant—as an opportunity for personal growth. Not that such people consciously sit down and tell themselves, "Now here is an opportunity for growth!" Rather, it is that such people have developed coping mechanisms that make it possible for them not only to deal with difficult life situations but also to gain new understandings and strengthen their spiritual foundations.

Even in the case of terminal illness—certainly the ultimate challenge to a person's emotional and spiritual resources—the adaptive personality allows the illness to teach him or her to appreciate life and the beauty of the earth more than ever before. John Wayne, the story goes, was already very ill with advanced cancer when a friend came to visit him one morning and commented, "What a beautiful day!" John Wayne replied, "Every day you wake up is a beautiful day!"

Or, to cite Dennis Potter again, "We tend to forget that life can only be defined in the present tense. It *is* and it is *now* only . . . Things are both more trivial than they ever were and more important than they ever were—and the difference between the two doesn't matter. But the *nowness* of everything is absolutely wondrous . . . The fact is that if you see the present tense, boy! can you see it, and boy! can you celebrate it."[11]

Another example comes to mind of how the adaptive personality is able to turn dire adversity into an opportunity for emotional and spiritual growth. The prize-winning German film maker Doris Doerrie described in a press interview how, just before filming of *Nobody Loves Me* was to start, her husband was diagnosed with liver cancer. "My husband was undergoing chemo while we were shooting," she said, "and we had people who were HIV positive in the crew. And in a funny way, it changed the way we all worked together. Everything became very light and very easy and funny. Once you realize that we are all dying together, once we really understand this, it's much easier to give up hatred and racism and egotism. It does make life more joyful."[12]

As we said in the beginning of this chapter, our emotions and our whole mentality, how well we deal with the stress that comes our way, and how adaptive and flexible we are, have a profound effect on our immune system, our endocrine system, and our neurological system. Attempts at life extension that focus exclusively on physical factors, without equal attention to our mental, emotional, and spiritual well-being, are therefore doomed to fall short. That, unfortunately, is a point often lost in our frantic striving for more and better antioxidants, youth hormones, genetic engineering, attempts at human cloning, and all the rest. For what good would it do to extend life that has no meaning and no promise of transcendence?

NOTES

1. *The New York Times* (International Edition). 6 Oct. 1995.
2. *Amer. J. Publ. Health.,* 1991; 81:719–24.
3. *Nature,* vol. 351, June 6, 1991; 429.
4. Eysenck, H. J. *Smoking, Personality, and Stress—Psychosocial Factors in the Prevention of Cancer and Coronary Heart Disease.* NY: Springer-Verlag, 1991; 89.
5. As reported at the American Psychiatric Convention, San Francisco, May 1993.
6. *The New York Times,* 15 Oct. 1995.
7. *The New York Times,* 5 Aug. 1997.
8. *The New York Times,* 14 Aug. 1997.
9. *The New York Times,* 30 July 1994.
10. Blum, David. Bucking the Biggest Odds of All. *The New York Times,* 19 June 1994.
11. *The New York Times,* 30 July 1994.
12. *The New York Times,* 29 Oct. 1995.

Part Nine

Vital Medical Alternatives

We feel compelled to inform you of some vital but little known facts concerning medical alternatives that can make a big difference—in fact, they can, without exaggeration, mean the difference between life and death.

One of these medical alternatives concerns a totally different way of using cancer chemotherapy. We hope to show you that with cancer the choice is not just between the orthodox medical route, on the one hand, and an "alternative" one, on the other hand, that shies away from anything "medical." Rather, there is a third option—a more ingenious and more benign approach to cancer therapy—as you will see from our interviews with oncologist Robert A. Nagourney, M. D., director of the Institute for Rational Therapeutics in Long Beach, California.

Another medical alternative concerns a knifeless way of

performing prostate surgery, rather than the usual, bloody and painful surgical removal of the prostate. You will learn about it from our interview with Giovanna Casola, M. D., of the Medical Center, University of California, San Diego.

Lastly, we will tell you of certain adjunct nutritional means of dealing with benign (nonmalignant) prostate enlargement that can render medical treatment more effective and produce faster results.

Chapter 51

Personalized Chemotherapy

While convalescing from his colon resection at Long Beach Memorial Hospital, Eberhard had almost daily conversations with Dr. Nagourney, an oncologist and professor of medicine, University of California, Irvine, when he stopped by on his rounds. That is how we learned a lot about his completely different approach to cancer and cancer therapy.

What he was doing seemed so much more logical and superior to cancer therapy "as we know it," and the patients he was telling us about were apparently doing a lot better than with standard chemotherapy. The reason for his success sounded logical enough, as he explained it to us then, at Eberhard's bedside: not every breast cancer, or colon cancer, or prostate cancer, or whatever, is alike, or will behave alike. Although they have enough characteristics in common to be labeled as this or that kind of cancer, in actual fact, one person's cancer cells may react very differently to the same chemotherapy drugs from those of another patient with an identical cancer.

It follows that you cannot treat every breast cancer, or colon cancer, or lung cancer, or whatever, alike either. But how can the doctor know with what drugs to treat a particular patient's unique cancer cells? The disconcerting truth is, your doctor really does not know and cannot know. All that the doctor knows is that, *on average,* a certain kind of cancer—say, estrogen-dependent breast cancer—responds best to such-and-such a combination of chemotherapy drugs. Let's say 70% of such cancers do respond favorably to this kind of therapy. But what if the patient happens to be among the unlucky 30% whose cancer cells refuse to act like well-behaved, "average" cancer cells?

What doctors do in that case is try to see if higher and higher and more and more toxic doses of the drugs will force the cancer into remission (what Dr. Nagourney calls "the sledgehammer approach"). But despite such risky treatments, quite often the resistant cancer cells won't oblige and die, no matter how hard they get hit with the toughest cancer drugs. In the process, the healthy cells get injured as well, the immune system is damaged, and the cancer patient becomes vulnerable to yeast or bacterial infections, not unlike the case with AIDS patients. And, like them, cancer patients who have been unsuccessfully treated with the wrong chemotherapy drugs often succumb to these treatment-caused infections, rather than to the cancer itself.

For that reason, Dr. Nagourney subjects every patient's biopsied cancer cells to different kinds of chemotherapy drugs in his own high-tech laboratory. If a patient's cancer cells don't respond to the standard chemo drugs, "one has to do a little creative thinking," Dr. Nagourney says. "Perhaps they will respond to something completely 'off the wall,' or to some different combination of drugs that no one else has thought of trying."

That's where Dr. Nagourney's true genius comes in. He is

as much of a brilliant biochemist as a practical clinician, and you've got to be both to succeed in what he is doing.*

After Eberhard's recovery we visited Dr. Nagourney's laboratory, where he let us see with our own eyes—looking through a high-powered microscope at a patient's cancer cells—how a commonly used combination of cancer drugs had not touched the patient's cancer cells at all, while another, less common combination had killed them off promptly.

At the same time, we were very upset to realize how many cancer patients are being mistreated daily with the wrong drugs. The shocking truth is that cancer patients are not given the same benefit of drug testing that is basic procedure for infectious diseases. People would be outraged if a doctor just used guesswork to prescribe an antibiotic for someone's life-threatening infection, without first determining by a laboratory test what drug is most effective in this particular case. But that is exactly what is going on in the case of cancer; the same drugs are used, pretty much, for everyone. Patients are constantly treated with drugs that only *in theory* have the best chance of working, but not necessarily in actual practice.

Part of the trouble is that most cancer specialists either don't know about the kind of laboratory test Dr. Nagourney is using, or are prejudiced against it. (There was another type of test, some years ago, that also was supposed to show which chemo-drugs were best for any patient's particular cancer cells. But it didn't work, and ever since there has been much skepticism in the medical community against all such testing.)

Whatever the reasons for the "cancer establishment" to ignore this important opportunity of finding out what the individual patient's particular cancer cells are most sensitive to, the

*In September 1996, ABC's evening news anchor, Peter Jennings, devoted a segment of his weekly program *Health Solutions*, to Dr. Nagourney's sophisticated ways of finding the right cancer drugs for individual patients. Video tapes or transcripts of this broadcast can be obtained from Dr. Nagourney's laboratory, Rational Therapeutics, Inc., 3601 Elm Ave., Long Beach, CA 90807 (562-989-6455).

result is that doctors don't set aside any cancer cells from biopsies for such testing. In consequence, patients are routinely exposed to highly toxic drugs, without any prior assurance that they are the right ones to use.

These are the reasons why we felt conscience-bound to inform you, the reader—whether you are a person with cancer, or not—that there is a better way, if need be, of treating cancer with chemotherapy. For that reason, we spent many hours interviewing Dr. Nagourney to let him explain his very different views of cancer and how to treat it more effectively.

Chapter 52

Another View of Cancer: Interview I with Robert A. Nagourney, M.D.

Q: Let us start with what may be a dumb question, What is cancer all about? In other words, what really is this terrible, much feared thing called cancer?

Dr. N.: That's not a dumb question at all. Most people would answer that cancer is a disease in which certain cells grow too much. By growing too much, cancers then invade normal tissues, prevent normal body functions, and ultimately overtake the host.

Q: But that's not the way you look at it, is it?

Dr. N.: Well, I think this whole concept of cancer needs to be reexamined. In fact, it may need to be entirely abandoned.

Q: With all due respect, that doesn't appear as obvious as it seems to be to you.

Dr. N.: I am just questioning. What if we were to assume that cancers, instead of growing too much, die too little? By looking at cancer as an immortality problem rather than a proliferation problem, we would begin to have a whole new way of looking at things. This, in scientific terms, is known as a paradigm shift, in which you reexamine data in a wholly new way and analyze everything again that you thought you'd already analyzed.

Q: But what does that mean in practical terms?

Dr. N.: All right, let's examine this proposition and consider several further questions. The most obvious thing to ask ourselves is, "If the main problem with cancer cells is that they grow too much, why is it that cancer drugs that are effective at stopping growth don't cure cancer?" Perhaps cancer cells don't actually "grow" more than normal cells; but just don't die the way normal cells do. In other words, if you view cancer as an immortality problem, then, perhaps, you begin to get to the root of the problem.

Q: But how would it affect actual cancer therapy?

Dr. N.: First of all, it will change cancer therapy from being guided by how the *majority* of patients react to cancer drugs to how the *individual* patient reacts to the drugs. That's why, for the past twelve years, my colleagues and I here at Rational Therapeutics have been using a seventy-two hour assay, or test, with the patient's own cancer tissue, measuring not what stops cancer cells from growing, but what actually kills them.

Q: Why is it that this isn't done routinely by every oncologist in the land?

Dr. N.: The answer is that what we're doing runs head-on against medical dogma.

Q: What dogma?

Dr. N.: The dogma is that tissue cultures of cancer cells don't work. Some years ago there was a laboratory assay called the stem-cell or clonogenic assay. The concept was that if you could add drugs to the proliferating (growing) population of cancer cells and prevent proliferation, or growth, then you could prevent the major danger of tumors—uncontrollable growth. That was the target of the assay.

The problem was that the assay didn't work. There were

a variety of reasons why it didn't work. One of them was that they were trying to assess the reactions of the most sensitive population of cells. Proliferative cells are the most sensitive to their environment. When you introduce any drug whatsoever into this population of cells, you begin to see effects that may not play out in a largely defended, more differentiated tumor mass, which constitutes 99.9% of the tumor. So this whole effort was programmed to fail from the very beginning.

What happened then is that after several years of testing with an assay that didn't work, the entire field of primary culture cancer cell testing was thrown out. It is as if you'd let the failed Ford Edsel destroy the whole automobile industry in perpetuity.

That's exactly what happened. There should, today, be a thriving field of laboratory investigation of human tumors, but instead we allowed this single failure to put an end to all of this work. It is only after a decade of our vigorous arguing that investigators—mostly in Europe—have taken up the banner and are now leading the field in an area of investigation that we developed.

When one examines the best laboratory tests for cancer today, it appears that the best assays are not those measuring growth inhibition, or DNA synthesis, or clonogenic cell growth. Instead, the best assays seem to be cell kill assays. In other words, tests that measure the ability of drugs to kill cells give you a lot of information about cancer.

That raises a very interesting question: What is it that dying cancer cells are telling you?

At the time we began working with these assays, we weren't actually aware of the implications of our work. We just thought we were looking at a relatively simple, relatively easily calibrated, rather technically attractive approach to the measurement of cell injury due to different kinds of chemotherapy exposure.

We have now come to realize that we lucked into a field that has now become the preeminent area of investigation of human cancer—the investigation of *apoptosis*.

Apoptosis, coming from the Greek term for the seasonal

loss of leaves from trees, is actually the process by which biological systems shed nonviable cells by killing them off and extracting from them what they need. With the trees the food stuff is removed from the dying leaves and the leaves drop off, having no more real value to the tree. The same way, body cells are eliminated from the body when the body no longer needs them. For instance, we are both male and female as embryos, and it is decided early in gestation whether you are going to be male or female. The body simply reabsorbs the opposite sex's counterparts, once the decision is made. The same way with webbing between your fingers, and so on.

So, in that regard, reabsorption of tissue is a natural process in the body. The body will actually reabsorb cancers. By assessing in the laboratory what drug is likely to induce apoptosis in these particular cancer cells, I can expose the patient to relatively nontoxic drugs, and when the drugs arrive at the tumor, their selective antitumor toxicity results in tumor cell death, but the cell death is *apoptotic*, not *necrotic*—the difference being that in apoptosis the cells are not totally destroyed, blown up, as it were, but reabsorbed into the body.

Q: That seems to need some more explanation.

Dr. N.: There are three ways in which injured cells can respond to environmental stress:

The first mechanism is a viability response wherein the cells produce stress proteins, heat-shock proteins, and other substances that will actually block the damage, dampen the fire, and allow the body and the cell to continue to live.

If the injury is more severe and the cell is clearly not viable, it's almost as if there is a program within the cell that tells it, "You're not going to be able to survive this injury, but if we work fast we can salvage parts of you before you die." It's like with an old car—it may no longer run, but some of its components may become valuable spare parts for other old cars. When a fifty-five Buick, like mine, has gotten to a point beyond repair, you have two options—let it rust out and become a piece of junk, or salvage anything that's still useful to people who need parts for other vintage Buicks.

In the same regard, if your body has the opportunity, it will actively absorb the tissue components of the dying cell and distribute them to other cells in the neighboring area that are in need of them.

In contrast, the process by which cells are totally lost is *necrosis*. That happens when the injury is so severe that nothing remains useful, like when cells are burned by fire, destroyed by acid, and so on. There is no reabsorption and no opportunity to use the components. In this case, the cell dissolves, or it bursts open and spreads into its immediate environment with all its enzymatic materials that induce inflammation, and the patient gets very sick.

In cancer, cells have escaped the natural senescence process—in other words, they have failed to age. Normal cells are supposed to live for only a period of months, die, and be replaced by other cells. But there is no net gain. If you have too many cells growing, before other cells can die, as in cancer, then you have an accumulation of excessive cells.

That's been the entire focus of cancer research—how can we prevent this growth? But the other side of the equation is inadequate death—the inadequate removal of tissue to make room for other cells. So we have to ask, why are cancer cells not dying? What is the metabolic counterpart to immortality? At what site in the cell is the time clock set and reset? These are the questions that need to be reexamined.

So we know today hundreds and thousands of genes, but we do not understand the simplest process by which an abnormal gene confers a growth potential on a cell. Or how an abnormal gene can result in the cell's failure to die.

However, the most important question today—from a practical, clinical point of view—is not *how* cancer got to be, but *what is it*? To me, as a clinician dealing with patients who are suffering and dying from cancer, it is less important to know which defective genes predisposed them to the disease than what is happening to them when tissue is growing in their livers, their lungs, or wherever. I would like to know what confers these immortality advantages to cancer cells.

That is why, in our laboratory, we are examining cancer from real people because, in my opinion, cancer from people is where the answer is. It may be very seductive and very easy to use cell lines, which are immortalized tissues growing forever in test tubes. Or you can use animal models. But the trouble is these only give you answers to artifical kinds of cells and about tumors in animals. They do not tell you very much about what is happening to patients when tissue is growing somewhere in their bodies.

What we need to get down to is figure out what is going on in the patient's liver or kidney or bone marrow that confers these immortality advantages to cancer cells. It is probably simple. With the sophisticated methodologies available to us today, the questions that scientists like Otto Warburg and Szent-Györgyi were posing in the 1930s and 1940s are answerable.

The reality unfortunately is that we are getting absolutely nowhere in understanding and treating cancer. We are just spinning our wheels.

That even goes for many, perhaps most, clinical trials. If you carefully examine the mechanism by which we study cancer and treat cancer today, you will find that a substantial number of clinical trials have no therapeutic intent. Very often there isn't even the pretense that we are going to help anybody.

For example, there was a drug, developed in the 1970s by a group at M. D. Anderson Cancer Center, that was thought to have anticancer activity. So it went into clinical trials and 2,748 patients, if I remember correctly, received it. The response rate was 2.7%, and almost all of these few responders were hemologic tumors—leukemias and lymphomas. Yet they continued to treat pancreas, head and neck, lung cancer, and so on, with this drug.

In fact, 168 patients received this drug for small cell lung cancer and zero responded. Now if you were patient 168, wouldn't you want to say, "Wait a minute, doc, is it really necessary that I be number 168 when there have been zero hits for 167 at bats?"

Q: No wonder so many cancer patients are looking for

help outside of mainstream medicine. Is there anything to improve patients' chances of survival within mainstream medicine?

Dr. N.: Sure. A lot can be done, for instance, to increase the effectiveness of some cancer drugs. Some time ago, I made a series of experiments to determine whether or not a chemotherapy drug called nitrogen mustard had any interaction with alpha-interferon.* As a completely unrelated comparison I used 5 FU (5-fluorouracil), an antimetabolite,† which is also a popular chemotherapy drug.

Frankly, I had not expected any interaction between alpha-interferon and 5 FU. But the two drugs not only interacted, there was enormous superadditivity. I have been able to put this little discovery to good use for several of my patients.‡

The most important practical point I'd like to make, however, is the fact that since you can measure cell death *in vitro* in our ninety-six-hour assay, you can determine whether patients are going to get better or not. What we've come to realize is that response of cancer patients to chemotherapy is not the function of the drugs used, but a function of the patient. Patients are biologically predetermined to be relatively responsive or not, because their cancers are either killable or not.

With available therapeutic agents—drugs—we are either able to unlock the process of cell senescence and cell death, or we aren't. If the patient doesn't respond to treatment, we've either been using the wrong drug, or the patient is constitutionally unresponsive to chemotherapy, period.

But that is something we don't like to face. So we try using megadoses of very toxic drugs, or we use "heroic" treatments

*Interferons are natural substances produced in response to infections. They have been created artificially by recombinant DNA technology in an attempt to control cancer.

†Antimetabolites refer to a family of antitumor drugs that resemble normal vitamins or building blocks of metabolism. They bind to the tumor's enzymes and chemical pathways. The tumor cells "think" they are getting the real vitamin and starve to the point where they can't grow or multiply.

‡Woolley, P. V., et al. *Proc. ASCO,* 1984.

like bone marrow transplants to make the patient respond. But what happens when you use very, very, very high doses of chemotherapy? You've moved out of the *apoptosis* pattern of stress in which cancer cells die and are reabsorbed by the body, into the stress leading to the *necrosis* pattern, wherein the patient's cancer cells explode like hand grenades, and the patient becomes desperately ill. And at the end of the day, if the patient gets over it at all, you may or may not have achieved a response, but you definitely have added twenty years to that patient's aging process. The oxidative stresses that people are put through by giving them these megadoses of chemotherapy age them dramatically.*

All of this could be avoided, if doctors and cancer researchers would only stop denying the obvious. Which is that when a cancer cell is exposed to a certain cancer drug in the test tube and dies, that patient is going to get better. In that case, you could, nine times out of ten, treat the patient even with a different drug, and he or she would still get better, because the cancer cell was killable. Not because the drug was so good, but the cancer was sensitive.

The cancer often isn't just sensitive to one particular drug, but to many drugs, because it is the cancer cell itself—the biological phenomenon of the cancer cell—that is the determining factor for the outcome—not some mysterious pharmaceutical factor, or some point on a dose-response curve—finding the optimal dose. This means people with cancer fall into two categories—relatively responsive and unresponsive.

When you realize this, and realize cancer cells live or die from the right drugs, like the right keys fitting into locks, and you find the right key for that patient's particular lock by doing a prior assay to guide you to the right drugs, then you no longer have to bludgeon the door open with a sledgehammer. And it

*As oncologist Dr. Charles Simone points out, the least doctors should do to minimize the impact of megadose chemotherapy or radiation therapy is to put patients on a protective vitamin/antioxidant regimen—but that, again, is a matter of controversy within the professional community.

certainly is a sledgehammer effect when doctors rev up the doses to as much as ten times as high as what is considered the lethal level.

If you're the patient and your body is the recipient of this kind of sledgehammering, wouldn't you prefer to have someone gently open the door to your cancer with the right key, rather than sledgehammering his way in? That's why it's so important for people with cancer to realize that—contrary to current medical opinion—there exists a laboratory test that can predict in advance whether the patient's cancer is sensitive to drugs and which drugs are the best keys to fit this particular cancer.

It may not be that, with the 1.1 million cancers this year and the sixty-plus FDA-approved drugs, there is a drug for every patient. We may not have a chemotherapy for every patient. But I'll bet you, there is a patient for every drug!

Q: Can you think of a case history that would illustrate the point?

Dr. N.: Well, I recently had a nineteen-year-old Honduran patient. That young fellow achieved a complete remission on corticosteroids after failing every known poison. And the reason he did so is that it was evident from our *in vitro* assay that exposing this patient's cancer cells to the corticosteroids induced apoptosis. They were the right key, and all the other, highly toxic drugs were the wrong keys. And even though they were sledgehammers, they couldn't sledgehammer open this guy's cancer lock.

But with the right key, the corticosteroids which we identified in the test tube, we induced this young fellow into remission, without his ever suffering a single side effect from the treatment. His body simply absorbed the tumor. And it was two kilograms!

This patient came with a white cell count of 375,000. He dropped his white count in five days of therapy with dexamethazone—a corticosteroid—to zero, without any toxicity at all. The process of apoptosis was induced, just as indicated beforehand by the laboratory observations which showed that this patient was sensitive to corticosteroids. His cancer cells had retained the pathway to death, and all we did was unlock it.

The sad part about it is that this young patient was a graduate of a major medical center's heavy-duty sledgehammer chemotherapy. He was so battered by prior chemotherapy that his bone marrow, once completely cleared of leukemia, had no residual normal cells to replenish his immune system. So he died from a fungal infection, as frequently happens with AIDS. His autopsy was aleukemic—no leukemia. On steroids alone! And there was no damage to his bone marrow, because dexamethazone does not hurt the bone marrow. And if someone had walked up to this poor guy the first day and put him on something like corticosteroids, maybe he would still be alive today.

Q: Perhaps it would be useful if you could explain, very briefly, how standard cancer therapy is practiced by mainstream oncology today.

Dr. N.: The current concept of cancer therapeutics is basically an algorithm, or a procedure for solving a mathematical problem. The patient appears with an abnormality—let's say, a lump in the neck. From there begins a whole decision tree. Number one: lump in the neck, benign or malignant? You make a decision, wait two weeks for improvement or growth, and if after two weeks the lump in the neck has gotten bigger, then we probably are looking at cancer. Number two: you do a biopsy, which allows you to examine histologically whether this is a cancer or a noncancerous growth. The biopsy shows that it is cancer. Number three: now you have to say what kind of cancer. It looks like lymphoma. Okay, what kind of lymphoma? Decision number four: Hodgkin's disease or non-Hodgkin's disease? It's non-Hodgkin's disease. Decision number five: what type of non-Hodgkin's disease? Is it B-cell follicular, or not? It's a B-cell follicular lymphoma.

Now, in traditional oncology, you treat this cancer with any one of a number of drugs or combinations of drugs. You choose drug X or combination XYZ. Why do you choose it? Because fifty years of chemotherapeutics have told you that *on average*, this kind of cancer responds to drug X or combination XYZ in 40, 50, or 60% of cases, and these people get better.

This is based on the fundamental idea, shared by most oncologists, that all cancers are created equal and that the treatment you are recommending is the best treatment for this patient, because you assume that the patient will behave like the average patient. The problem is, there is no "average patient." Conventional cancer therapeutics take statistics like that and force them onto patients. But, in real terms—as far as the individual patient is concerned—we just don't have a 37% response rate, patients don't get 82% remissions. They are either in remission or not. And our job is to make a decision, right up front, about who is going to go into remission and with what drug, and who isn't.

We just have to throw off this "average patient" illusion, because it is just not going to apply to patients on an individual basis. Instead, patients need to be given the respect of having their own therapy—not some "average therapy" that may not apply to them at all. After all, they wear their own shoe size, their own dress or suit size, they wear their own prescription eye glasses. Why shouldn't patients be entitled to get the kind of chemotherapy that is most likely to cure them?

Let's face it—more often than not, the current process of cancer therapy isn't working. There is no more glaring example of that than lymphoma itself. In 1993, there was a study published in *The New England Journal of Medicine,* in which Richard Fisher and his co-authors compared treatments for lymphoma. Now, if there is any single cancer in the world that we should have been able to treat, it is lymphoma. This is a disease of B-cells, which are highly selective for sensitivity to treatment. These are the cells that disappear if you are exposed to too much sunlight or any amount of radiation. These are the cells that, when they become malignant, are highly sensitive to treatment. We should be curing many, if not most, of these people.

Instead, we have been forcing patients into this "average patient" paradigm, and we haven't been able to cure a high percentage of lymphomas. Clinical oncology has failed to take into consideration the reality that some patients' cancer cells weren't listening. They were just not going to benefit from this "average patient" approach.

As a response to such a high failure rate, we keep coming up with increasingly intense and increasingly complex regimens, consisting of more and more drugs, until we have some drug combinations that have eleven different chemotherapies. But when we get down to the real world of testing one combination against another, it turns out they are all exactly the same. They all yield the same level of durable remission at a three-year analysis—although some of the regimens are incredibly toxic. The only statistically significant difference between regimens was that the more intensive regimens had induced more serious toxicities and more deaths.

Look at the whole statistical foundation of what is happening with this sort of approach to cancer therapy. Let's say, we've got one hundred patients being treated in this manner. We know from clinical experience that out of that one hundred patients, seven will die because the combination was too toxic. Twenty-five people will have responses, and ten of them are going to be cured.

So the statistics say, there is 7% mortality, a 75% failure rate, and you only get 10% out of the one hundred cured. What these statistics tell you is that this kind of treatment doesn't work. But ask Mr. Jones, who is alive today because he was one of the 10% who got cured, if it didn't work!

The point is, while we continue to act as if cancer patients all respond the same, and combination treatments or single drug treatments are going to give the same relative outcomes in each patient, we are going to come to the conclusion that treating the hundred people wasn't worth it. But you tell me, if only one patient out of the one hundred was cured, wouldn't that patient insist that his treatment had worked? Any patient who got better with chemotherapy would argue to his death that he is alive today only because of it.

So, when people tell me that chemotherapy doesn't work, it's too toxic, it poisons people, the statistics aren't any good, I say, wait a minute—chemotherapy works for whom it works. Our job as responsible doctors is to find the responders before ever starting therapy. And to find what they respond to best. And if the patient doesn't respond to most anything in our usual assortment of cancer drugs, we've got to be inventive and throw other, unconventional drugs at his cancer cells in the test tube to find one to which they may be sensitive.

If this kind of laboratory investigation is done first, I can show you unequivocally that cancer chemotherapy works. And often with greatly reduced toxicity and side effects. Your hair doesn't necessarily have to fall out, vomiting and malaise may be unnecessary, because if we find the right drug, a lower dose can often still get the same results. We've seen that in case after case in our own laboratory, when we have had a chance to do a primary tissue culture assay and the treatment is based on the assay results. To my mind, that's what rational cancer chemotherapy is all about.

As I said before, we have to stop worrying why cancer cells keep growing and focus on why they're not dying. We've got to measure their death in the test tube. And if the cancer cells die in the test tube, they'll also die in the patient. That's what we have been seeing with our primary tissue assay for the past ten or twelve years.

I have a woman patient in my practice now who appeared with pancreatic cancer. I got a piece of tissue right out of her neck and it showed it was metastatic. This lady was as good as dead; it's rare that pancreatic cancer goes into remission. But to our delight she tested sensitive to a certain chemotherapy. She bounced into remission with two cycles of relatively nontoxic therapy. She is now nearly one year posttreatment and is working and enjoying life. Even if her cancer should come back some time in the future—remember, she was metastatic!—we bought her some precious time, and have done so without making her suffer.

Q: Did she have previous chemotherapy?

Dr. N.: No! That's the trick. I've got to get people before they ever get poisoned with drugs their cancer is not sensitive to anyway, but which only make them more resistant.

But sometimes one can get almost miraculous results, using the primary tissue assay, even in cases that have already been treated unsuccessfully. For instance, another recent case of mine involved a fifty-eight-year-old patient from Israel with recurrent ovarian cancer. She had stage four adenocarcinoma of the ovary and had been given standard chemotherapy, prior to being referred to me. Regrettably, however, the clinical course was one of progressive pain and demonstrable increases in CA 125, a test that is elevated in cancers of the ovaries and uterus. Thereupon she had been put on Taxol, but, after receiving four cycles of it, was found resistant to this drug.

Fortunately, however, our short-term suspension culture assay revealed that her cancer was responsive to the experimental and little-known drug gemcitabine. She has been undergoing chemotherapy with this drug, plus cisplatin, and has been responding very well, exceeding our fondest expectations. In fact, she improved so much during this "off-brand" chemotherapy that she was able to return to Israel for the remainder of the therapy.

We could not help but think of poor Gilda Radner, the television comedienne, who also was resistant to all of the commonly used chemotherapy drugs. For years her doctors literally tortured her, as she tells in *It's Always Something,* with more and more toxic cancer drug combinations. Unlike the Israeli woman Dr. Nagourney was talking about, she did not have the good fortune of coming to the attention of an oncologist like him, who, by testing her cancer tissue, might have discovered another "off-brand" drug that could have saved her life.

Other, similar cases come to mind—for instance, the still more recent cancer death of the singer Nancy LaMott, whose cancer was also unresponsive to the usual cancer drugs. She, too, might have been cured, if a prior test had indicated that her cancer was vulnerable to some little-used drug. But, whether the person in question is famous or not, we find it extremely disturbing that so many people have to die for what seems to be nothing more than medical prejudice.

Chapter 53

"How Would You Have Treated Jackie O.?" Interview II with Robert A. Nagourney, M.D.

Shortly after Jackie Onassis died in New York of a very aggressive type of lymphoma, we met again with Dr. Nagourney. With her death fresh in our minds, we interviewed him—whom we knew to have a very different "take" on cancer—about what he might have done, had he been her oncologist.

This is what he said:

The closest example I can come to Jackie O. is a patient I'm currently managing named Eric. At the age of thirty-one he suddenly felt a lump on his neck. He suspected it was cancer, but he had no medical insurance and no regular employment. However, he had the good fortune of having a girlfriend with a little money and a good heart, who decided he should see a cancer specialist and she would help him pay for it. But the only oncologist they knew was one who had specialized in recent years in breast cancer. Realizing that it probably was lymphoma, that doctor suggested that he see me.

So this patient arrived at my office for an evaluation. I found that he had lymphadenopathy (disease of the lymph nodes) in several parts of the body. He had night sweats and constitutional symptoms—symptoms affecting the whole body.

I suggested he needed a formal staging, which consisted of a CAT scan and other investigations. I also explained that he would need a biopsy to establish the architecture and the appearance of the tumor and provide cancer cells for the assay I use to determine what kind of chemotherapy would be best in any particular patient's case.

The trouble was that all of that involved quite a bit of money and, remember, this guy had no insurance, practically no money of his own, and was totally dependent on his girlfriend's good will and limited funds. The CAT scan would cost in excess of $1,000, and the cost of bilateral bone marrow biopsy another $500; to undergo surgical biopsy of the tumor could cost another $2,000. I had to tell him that, before spending $2,000 to $3,000 per cycle of chemotherapy—which could add up to $25,000 to $50,000, or more—he would spend $5,000 to $10,000, just for the preliminary investigations.

I therefore suggested that he find an institution such as the University of Southern California or City of Hope, a large California cancer treatment center, with programs for poor patients with cancer, to see if he could get all of this done free.

He set about looking into that, but returned to me the following week and said he had carefully considered everything and arrived at certain conclusions. He would be happy to receive further work-up and chemotherapy at other institutions, but he'd prefer to first have me give him my best opinion, based upon my own primary tissue test, about the kind of therapy I considered best for him.

I therefore offered to get him fully staged as quickly and

cheaply as possible, and I donated a complete laboratory investigation of his responsiveness to various chemotherapies at my laboratory.

The patient underwent a surgical biopsy and complete staging, and I did bone marrow biopsies on him myself. They revealed, most regrettably, that he had a B-cell, intermediate grade, non-Hodgkin's lymphoma—stage four. That meant he had bone marrow involvement and extensive adenopathy throughout his abdomen.

The biopsy also provided me with ample tumor tissue for my series of chemotherapy sensitivity tests. Much to my dismay, they revealed that the patient was resistant to many standard cytotoxic drugs, that is, drugs toxic to the patient's cancer cells.

Eric meanwhile kept looking around for a place where he could get the chemotherapy, once I had found something that his particular cancer cells were sensitive to. It turned out that the only place willing to take him in was City of Hope.

So the patient went to City of Hope. Included with my referral were the results of all my laboratory investigations, recommending that instead of standard combination chemotherapy he required a certain chemotherapy drug, which was the only one his tumor cells were responsive to. I even sent them a copy of the abstract from the *Proceedings of the American Cancer Society,* describing this regimen.

Despite all this, the doctors at City of Hope put the patient on a standard combination chemotherapy and, of course, he failed to achieve a complete remission, despite the fact that normally intermediate grade, non-Hodgkin's lymphomas have between a 50 and 85% chance of doing so. For that reason alone, you'd think that the doctors at City of Hope would have been happy that I had been able to *a priori* identify a refractory patient for them, so they could change the therapy accordingly. But instead of listening to me, they wanted to go on with another standard combination therapy, even after this initial failure.

The patient returned to me, six months into therapy, now with at least one septic complication, telling me, "Doctor, I've had six cycles of this chemotherapy and I'm not in remission.

Now they want to do another biopsy. What do you advise me to do?"

I said, "Eric, I'm awfully sorry to hear about that and awfully sorry your doctors didn't take my recommendations to heart. But you must realize, I couldn't force them to follow my advice." But I called his doctor at City of Hope and asked why they wanted to rebiopsy him. She said, "Well, we want to confirm whether the histological diagnosis was accurate."

What they meant was, they wanted to see whether his tumor cells were really lymphoma, because only 15 to 20% of these patients fail to get full remission with standard chemotherapy. They didn't want to believe that this guy was one of those unfortunate exceptions, as my assay had clearly shown.

But as long as they wanted to do another biopsy, I told the patient, "Why don't you take the culture medium along with you and ask them to put a little of their tissue sample into it and send it to my lab at my expense, so I can do a second free assay to see whether anything has changed because of the chemotherapy."

The patient said, "Fine." He told the surgeon that I'd appreciate it if he'd do this when doing the biopsy. The surgeon said, "Fine." But the oncologist said, "No way. I'm not going to play ball with *in vitro* chemo-sensitivity tests, because they're all a bunch of hooey."

So the patient, realizing that he was up against a stone wall, returned to me and said, "How about if I pay to have the biopsy done here, since you are willing to run another assay, and send them, at City of Hope, a piece for their histological confirmation?" I said, "By all means."

I set him up for a biopsy with a surgeon here at the hospital. The sample was appropriately processed and returned to the City of Hope, while I had access to the tissue for my own assay. It revealed the following: the patient had become profoundly resistant to chemotherapies. Whatever he had been moderately sensitive to before, he was now utterly resistant to. The only effective drugs remaining were of a type not generally used with chemotherapy.

It so happened that, at this time, I had to attend an ASCO (American Society of Clinical Oncologists) meeting, and I deliberately sought out the patient's physician at City of Hope, and asked her to consider carefully our recommendation, instead of putting the patient on more standard chemotherapy and taking him into bone marrow transplant. I explained to her that our assay clearly showed that even the drug I had previously recommended, and which might have worked then, was no longer going to work. The patient had acquired resistance to everything. The tumor had become too smart for the drug. And I told her what I thought, based on our assay, was the only way to treat this patient now.

Instead of doing that, the people at City of Hope put this patient on another round of combination chemotherapy, which contained one of the drugs I had recommended, but also contained three very toxic compounds, including platinum. I had specifically tested the patient's tumor to see whether there was any positive interaction between the one possibly effective drug I would have used and platinum.

You see, for all we know, there may be synergy between them in some circumstances, but in his particular case there was no synergy at all. So there was absolutely no reason, in this case, to use platinum, one of the most toxic chemotherapy drugs there is.

On the other hand, there was a good possibility of putting this patient into partial or maybe complete remission by using only modest and relatively nontoxic doses of the one still positive drug I had discovered. I told them all this. But they utterly refused. Instead, they gave him two more cycles with the toxic combination therapy, followed by a bone marrow transplant, leaving him, after all this, still with persistent lymphoma.

By now he had been absolutely put through the wringer. He no longer had enough bone marrow reserve to go on to other chemotherapies. He looked terrible, and they said to him, in so many words, "Sorry, but you've failed. You no longer fit our protocol."

So the poor guy goes out and joins something called Jericho House, in the Duarte, California, area, near City of Hope. It is some kind of macrobiotic diet program. They eat only whole grains, organically grown vegetables, lots of soy products, and so on. No detergents, very organic life. And in six months he's no longer sick, in fact, he's pretty well.

But finally he begins to run into some problems. His lymph nodes in the left groin are beginning to swell. He's beginning to develop some spleen enlargement. His cancer is beginning to grow back. He goes back to City of Hope, but they tell him, there's not much we can offer you.

When he comes to see me he says, "I would like to go on nontraditional therapy." So I referred him to a man named Alan Kapuler, a microbiologist by profession, who seems to have managed his own lymphoma, using biological therapeutics and macrobiotic diet.

He talks to Dr. Kapuler and drives down to Tijuana, where he got injections of BCG (*Bacillus Calmette-Guerin*) and was put on a certain herbal mixture, the "Hoxsey tonic." But about six weeks later he comes back to see me, and he looks like death.

His left leg is three times the size of his right leg. His inguinal adenopathy (lymph gland enlargement in the groin) has grown to the point where it is almost palpable through his trousers. He's got a bright red, bloody left eye. His spleen and liver are almost palpable to the pelvic rim.

The patient's girlfriend turns to me, as he's dressing after the examination, and says, "Is this it? Is he dying?"

I said, "Honestly, I really don't know. I hope not."

So I go back to my old data on the patient, and I think, what is this guy sensitive to and what is he resistant to? The only thing I could remember that he was sensitive to were some antimetabolites, like cytosine arabinoside (ARA-C). But his platelet count is down to 14,000 by now* . . . I can't possibly put him on any cytotoxic drug, because his platelet count will go to zero and he'll have an intercranial bleed. So all I can do for the guy right now is put him on corticosteroids and hope

*Normal values for platelet count are 150,000–350,000.

that I can dampen the process long enough to stabilize him to get his bone marrow function up to a point where he will no longer be intolerant to mild cytotoxic drugs.

I put him on very high doses of prednisone. A week later his platelet count is still low, but his spleen is shrinking, his fevers have resolved, his left leg is improving, he's no longer bleeding into his eye, and he's feeling better.

A week goes by, and he is better still. Another week goes by, and he is increasingly better and better. I realize we've finally plateaued on the steroid benefit, and I start to taper him off slowly from the prednisone. But his platelet count never goes higher than 25,000.

Realizing it is now or never, I put him on what my test indicated was the best drug, ARA-C. Knowing, too, that "dose intensity"—higher and higher doses, another favorite of standard cancer therapy—was out of the question, I put him on only modest doses, to allow him to achieve response without significant toxicity. And, lo and behold, the patient responds, while we continue to taper him off his prednisone.

His spleen now goes back to almost normal, his lymph nodes in the groin return to normal, his left leg goes back to normal. But his platelet count remains low and he develops a dry cough and fever. I put him in the hospital, fearful that he has developed a septic process. A full week of evaluations, however, does not provide any evidence of the source of infection. Yet his lymphoma is clearly improving.

The day before I am to discharge him, his chest X ray reveals a fine grain interstitial infiltrate. I suspect he has *Pneumocystis carinii* pneumonia.* A pulmonary specialist sees him and confirms my preliminary diagnosis.

He's treated for it, and after he recovers I start him on the

***Pneumocystis carinii* pneumonia is now thought to be more of a fungal rather than bacterial or viral infection. Almost all patients with this disease have compromised immune systems. It is therefore frequently associated with cancer chemotherapy and AIDS.

next line of antimetabolites. This time, after the second cycle, the patient is achieving what may be a complete remission. Even after what happened to him at City of Hope and all the rest, we may still be able to save the life of this thirty-three-year-old father of a five-year-old child.

Now, to come back to your initial question, how would I have treated Jackie O.? The answer is that, since, like my patient, Eric, she did no longer respond to standard chemotherapy, I would, if possible, have run our assay on her cancer cells, to see whether there was any other drug her cancer might be responding to. I suppose, you wonder, Why didn't her own doctors—and I am sure she had the best doctors money can buy—do this? Well, I guess the answer is that different doctors may have different philosophical orientations, and many excellent physicians simply do not have much confidence in our laboratory tests. That's why I used my patient Eric's case, which highlights these differences in therapeutic approaches. If more patients become aware of these differences, they will be in a better position to make their own choices, as to what kind of treatment they want—which is exactly the reason I am taking time off giving interviews like this, including some with the news media.

Postscript

When all the hype about the new cancer drugs *angiostatin* and *endostatin* exploded in the popular media in the spring of 1998, we immediately called Dr. Nagourney to get his reaction. For to us, it seemed the media reaction was very overblown.

Dr. Nagourney thought so, too. He also confirmed the impressions we had gained a few years earlier when studying these same angiostatic substances—that is, those that inhibit the growth of new blood vessels. We had studied angiostatic substances in another context—shark cartilage, which contains varying amounts of them. For it had been assumed for some time—correctly, as it turned out—that they were responsible for whatever tumor-suppressing effect shark cartilage can produce.*

Dr. Nagourney pointed out that their effectiveness in inhibiting blood supply to tumors was also nothing new. "It has," he said, "over the past few years been demonstrated several times. But always only in mice—never, thus far, in humans. To infer from mice studies that these substances will be equally effective in humans represents a quantum jump into the still unknown.

"Sure, one hopes that it will turn out to be so. But we still don't know, and shouldn't set our hopes too high. A number of other substances, both pharmaceutical and natural, have also been effective in animals, but were disappointing when it came to humans. Nonetheless, this represents one of several new and promising directions in cancer research. Yet, the biology of metastasis—how do cells split off from tumors and migrate to different parts of the body?—not to mention the basic riddle—what makes cancer cells immortal?—remains as far from being solved as ever.

"We should also keep in mind," Dr. Nagourney continued, "that even if angiostatin and endostatin actually work also in humans in cutting off blood supply to tumors, it still does not mean, 'Now we can cure cancer.' Cancer is so darned smart, it might find a way of adjusting to this new challenge. That's the way it has been, every time we thought we had a cure for it.

"So, even in the best-case scenario, I'm sure we'll also need all kinds of other types of therapies, along with these blood vessel–inhibiting drugs, including the three standard weapons—surgery, chemotherapy, and radiation—in our cancer-fighting arsenal.

"Still, if angiostatin and endostatin turn out to work in humans, it would be a great boon in our continuing fight against

*Clinical studies with shark cartilage therapy, conducted in Cuba a few years ago, and involving actual cancer patients, did indeed show a certain beneficial but not very impressive tumor-inhibiting effect, the success rate being around 15%.

cancer. It would certainly enable us to reduce the dosages in chemotherapy, hopefully even below the already much lower-than-standard doses I am using in my own clinical practice. In some cases, we might even be able to use them alone, without any other therapies. But all of this is still unknown. We shall have to wait and see—and hope for the best."

Chapter 54

Prostate Cancer: A Different Approach: An Interview with Giovanna Casola, M.D.

On one of our frequent visits to southern California, we called a friend to see whether he had time to have dinner with us that weekend. To our shocked surprise, he said he unfortunately could not because he was going into the hospital the next day for some tests.

"What's the matter?" we asked anxiously, for he was one of our handful of closest friends. Only a short time ago, walking the beach with us, he had seemed in perfect health.

"Ah, well," he said in what seemed a deliberately casual tone of voice, "I've recently noticed some blood in my urine, and I'm going to have it checked out."

Of course, we knew that blood in the urine is always a serious matter. It could mean a really bad kidney or bladder infection. In a worst-case scenario it could be a symptom of advanced prostate cancer.

A week later, when the test results were in, it unfortunately turned out to be the latter and, apparently, a more aggressive case, because he was only in his early fifties. That sort of situation usually calls for radical prostatectomy (the complete removal of the whole prostate gland). Unless, that is, the cancer has already progressed beyond the prostate itself and invaded too much surrounding tissue, like the seminal vesicles and adjacent lymph nodes. In that case, the only thing—aside from chemotherapy—that can be done by standard medical practice is radiation therapy by external beam. (Implantation of radioactive seeds into the tumor wouldn't do in that case, because they cannot reach far enough into the surrounding tissue.)

At the time, as far as we were concerned, there seemed to be nothing else to do in a case like our friend's. Our ignorance about another, lesser known option—cryosurgery (from the Greek word element meaning cold)—can perhaps be excused, because many urologists, we found out, "don't believe in it," have "no confidence" in it, or have never given it much thought either.

One consequently finds few references to it in the medical literature, both of the scientific and popular variety.* Our friend, however, himself a medical doctor, had become aware of this option, looked at its pros and cons, and decided to be treated that way.

We became intrigued by this "new" way of treating prostate cancer, not only because of our friend, but also because radical prostatectomy is such "a severe and mean operation with many unpleasant side effects," as one prominent prostate cancer survivor and cancer research benefactor—billionaire Jon M.

*For instance, the otherwise excellent popular cancer book *Everyone's Guide to Cancer Therapy—How Cancer Is Diagnosed, Treated, and Managed Day by Day* (Sommerville House Books, 1991) does not even mention cryosurgery. Nevertheless, we highly recommend the book, because it contains much useful information about how cancer is diagnosed, "staged," and treated according to conventional medical practice. At the same time, however, we recommend, as a counterbalance, Ralph Moss's excellent book, *Cancer Therapy: A Guide to Alternative Cancer Therapies* (NY: Equinox Press, 1992/97).

Huntsman—put it.* An alternative medical treatment for radical prostatectomy is all the more important because the disease is as widespread among men, as breast cancer is among women.

Actually, cryosurgery, as we soon found out through a search of the medical literature, is not all that new, after all. The deliberate and controlled destruction of diseased tissue through freezing was already practiced in the mid-nineteenth century, when suitable refrigerants first became available. But liquid nitrogen, the refrigerant now used most in cryosurgery, was not available until the last few years of the nineteenth century.

Many readers have had experiences with liquid nitrogen treatments for skin cancer. But, obviously, that cannot be done with an internal organ like the prostate. For that a special apparatus, special instruments, and special techniques had to be invented.

The procedure itself is rather straightforward and, in principle, fairly simple: The patient undergoes anesthesia, either by spinal block or general anesthesia. Following that, five freezing "probes" (instruments resembling long syringes, but without needles and closed at the far end) are inserted into the perineum by an almost bloodless technique. (The pelvic area into which the freezing probes are inserted is located below the penis and scrotum and just above the rectum.)

To guide the doctor in inserting the probes so that they enter the prostate in the proper places, a "transrectal ultrasound probe" is inserted into the rectum. This enables the doctor to guide the probes by ultrasound to exactly the desired positions to freeze the entire prostate and some of the surrounding tissue. Only after that is liquid nitrogen forced, under pressure, into the five probes, which rapidly freeze the desired area with temperatures of at least −60 degrees centigrade (−140 degrees Fahrenheit).

*Jon M. Huntsman, survivor of both prostate and mouth cancer, founded and generously endowed the Huntsman Cancer Institute at the University of Utah. The Institute emphasizes early diagnosis and detection of cancer precursors, as well as early treatment.

At the same time, however, a flexible urethral warming device—really a modified catheter used in angioplasty*—is inserted through the penis to protect the urethra, testicles, and other tissues from the very low temperatures of the cryoprobes.

This, essentially, is the whole procedure, which lasts—much in contrast to radical prostatectomy—only a few minutes. However, the surgeons have to be very careful to prevent side effects, such as fistulas† in the perineum and the accidental freezing of areas, which could mean increased risk of incontinence and impotence.

That's why it is advisable, if one has decided to have this type of therapy, to have it done only in a medical center where the technique is practiced daily and the doctors' skills are finely honed. (The American hospitals that specialize in cryosurgery include the University of California Hospital, in San Diego, the Columbia-Presbyterian Hospital, in New York, and the Allegheny General Hospital, in Pittsburgh.) For it is on daily experience and almost virtuoso medical skills—much more so than in conventional surgery—that the final outcome of cryosurgery depends.

We are much indebted to our friend who underwent cryosurgery for introducing us to one of its most skilled practitioners, Giovanna Casola, M. D., associate professor of radiology at the Medical Center, University of California, in San Diego. We had a delightful luncheon interview with this dedicated doctor—an attractive, fortyish, Mediterranean-type woman. What she told us will give the reader a much better idea of what this promising, "alternative" prostate therapy is all about.

Following are excerpts from the interview:

Q: How do people find out about this almost "secret" technique of treating prostate cancer?

*Angioplasty refers to the surgical reconstruction of blood vessels, as for instance, in the repair of blocked coronary arteries.

†Fistula, in this case, would mean a holelike opening in the perineum through which body fluids from the operated on area would drain to the outside.

Dr. C.: People are searching for alternatives to conventional prostate cancer surgery because of its often serious side effects. They are looking at all kinds of options, and some of them somehow discover cryosurgery.

Q: What does conventional prostate cancer therapy consist of?

Dr. C.: Conventional therapy means, most of all, radical prostatectomy, or surgical removal of the entire prostate gland. Of course, there is also radiation therapy for some patients. By the time they come to us, they've already decided they don't like these options.

What usually happens is that the patient's family doctor, who sees there is a prostate problem of some kind, sends the patient to a urologist. If the urologist suspects prostate cancer, he sends the patient to an oncologist. And, nine times out of ten, the advice these patients are getting is to get a radical prostatectomy, or, if they are at more advanced stages, radiation.

Q: They are not told about cryosurgery?

Dr. C.: They are usually not told about cryosurgery. Most of them have to find out about it on their own. Sometimes, if there is too much risk with them getting conventional surgery, they may be told about cryosurgery.

Q: Do urologists know about cryosurgery?

Dr. C.: Some of them don't know much about it, and some of them don't take it seriously. However, in our medical community here in Southern California, they definitely do know. We've talked about it at urologists' meetings, given seminars, and so on. But that doesn't mean they all like it. Some of them have lost patients to us and they are not happy about that.

We must interrupt our interview to report on a strange coincidence that occurred just as we were discussing the attitudes of some urologists toward cryosurgery. Dr. Casola received an urgent phone call from the hospital, but it was not about a patient in trouble, as we had thought. Instead, it was to tell her that the FDA had just withdrawn its previous approval of the urethral warming device that prevents healthy tissue from being damaged by freezing. No explanation was offered for this sudden reversal, and there seemed no logical reason for it.

The serious part, as Dr. Casola explained, is that you cannot do cryosurgery of the prostate without protecting the rest of the urogenital area from below-zero cold. So, without the urethral warming device, no more prostate cryosurgery. One may therefore be justified to think of the possibility that this reversal of the FDA's prior approval of the warming device could have been due less to genuine concern about the device's actual safety than to the influence of powerful special interests, intent on killing a competitive procedure.

Dr. Casola, however, assured us that she and her colleagues had already worked out a backup technique in case the urethral warming device should ever fail them. In other words, they would be able to substitute for the capriciously banned device and keep right on performing safe and effective prostate cryosurgery.

To return to our interview:

Q: It must take a lot of courage, Dr. Casola, for a patient to opt for cryosurgery when major medical opinion either ignores cryosurgery or recommends radical surgery or radiation therapy instead.

Dr. C.: Yes, the patient who comes to us is going against the system. It's a very difficult thing to do as a patient. He's got to be strongly motivated. But I am sure, the more this gets written about and talked about, the more patients will be asking for it. It's sort of the rebels right now who are opting for it. They are taking a lot of responsibility for themselves. On the other hand, patients who are referred to us by urologists in this area are routinely given that option.

Q: At your hospital, are you also doing radical prostatectomies?

Dr. C.: We are hardly doing radicals in our institution anymore.

Q: How about laser therapy?

Dr. C.: Laser therapy is being done not for prostate cancer but for prostatic hypertrophy (prostate enlargement).

Q: Do you talk with the patients about their feelings concerning their cancer?

Dr. C.: The truth is, a lot of patients don't like to talk very much about their prostate cancer.

Q: Any idea why that is so?

Dr. C.: Because it's like with breast cancer in women, only much worse. Maybe we are here more into what many men feel is the essence of manhood, of virility. So to admit something is wrong with the prostate, or you have had it removed . . . there's a stigma associated with it. It's not like saying, well, I've had some skin cancer. When it comes to the prostate, it's got something to do with men's whole self-esteem.

Q: What about group support?

Dr. C.: It would be a very good thing. But we don't have it at our hospital for prostate cancer yet. Besides, men differ from women in that respect. Women, in general, are more open to discussion, to expressing feelings, that sort of thing. Men, on the other hand, are suffering internally, on their own, but find it difficult to get in touch with their feelings, much less sharing them with others.

That's why I feel there is a very big need for that sort of thing—informal group therapy. The psychological part is so crucial. Medicine and technology can only go so far. The rest is the mind, how the patient looks at things. Yes, I would like to see something along the lines of group support and group discussion for prostate patients started at our hospital. Men with prostate cancer are sort of a forgotten group.

Q: Do you have patients from outside the United States coming to you for cryosurgery?

Dr. C.: At this point it is all American. The procedure is only done in the United States and England. In England they started working with cryosurgery in the 1950s.

Q: Is the technology for cryosurgery very expensive?

Dr. C.: Not really. The cryo-machine which delivers the

liquid nitrogen costs around $200,000. An ultrasound machine costs around $50,000.

Q: How expensive is it for the patient?

Dr. C.: Not so bad. The costs for the procedure are significantly reduced by the savings in hospital stay. About half of our patients come in the morning and leave at night. The other half leave the next morning. They are a little bit uncomfortable, but they are going home.

Q: How much discomfort is there?

Dr. C.: Well, they have a sore bottom for a few days, but they are getting pain medication. Aside from that, the most discomfort is connected with having to have a catheter in the urethra to drain their bladder, because it is hard to urinate right after cryosurgery. But after seven to ten days, most patients can urinate again on their own. Once the urine is clear and there are no longer blood clots in it, the catheter comes out.

Also, the patients are placed on antibiotics for about two weeks to avoid infection. The risk of infection is small, and if it occurs it usually is a urinary infection. About 5% get some urinary infection, despite the antibiotics. But they don't have to be in the hospital for that to be treated.

Q: What are some of the worst things that can happen with prostate cryosurgery?

Dr. C.: The biggest complaints are still related to urinary incontinence. Actually, we've had no patients with total urinary incontinence. We have patients with what is called "stress incontinence" or "urgency incontinence."

Q: Can you explain these terms a little more?

Dr. C.: "Stress incontinence" is when you may lose some urine, for instance, when you cough or sneeze . . . what most of us women have to live with anyway, over time. But in men it is normally very rare, so they don't accept it as well. "Urgency incontinence" means when you have to go to the bathroom, you really have to go!

Q: Just how frequent is this partial incontinence?

Dr. C.: I would say no more than 3 to 5% of patients experience it.

Q: How about impotence?

Dr. C.: That's a tough question to answer. Many of our patients were receiving hormone depletion therapy* before, so they are already impotent because of that.

With some of the older patients, their impotency rate from our procedure is very difficult to assess. They may have varying degrees of vascular disease. But with some patients it's hard to find out their preoperative potency status. They either don't answer the question on the medical history questionnaire, or they don't answer truthfully. It's hard to get straight answers.

Generally speaking, cryosurgery is much superior in that respect to radical prostatectomy or radiation. If you cut nerves, as in conventional radical surgery, those nerves are gone. It's usually the same with external beam radiation. On the other hand, if you only freeze nerves, the way we are doing, they can regenerate.

Q: How long does that take?

Dr. C.: It takes from six months to a year for nerves to regenerate. So, if the patient is impotent right after cryosurgery, we tell him he may become more potent after the nerves have regenerated. A lot depends on factors that have nothing to do with the procedure, like diet, lifestyle, smoking, vitamins, mental state, relationship with his partner, and all the rest.

The men's whole concept of sex enters into it. They may have blocked it out totally . . . the fear of not being able to have an erection. Many of them don't even want to think about it. That doesn't help the healing phase.

Q: What is the actual risk of impotence with cryosurgery?

Dr. C.: We are telling our patients that the risk is 50% impotence, period. That's high, but with radical surgery it's up

*Hormone depletion therapy refers to either one of two things: it can, but rarely does, mean removal of the testes. This will stop most androgen (male hormone) production, thereby depriving the prostate cancer of the hormone on which it "feeds" and thus slowing its growth. Since prostate cancer cells seem, however, to get inured, over time, to testosterone depletion, some oncologists are alternating cycles of testosterone depletion with cycles of testosterone replacement.

to 70%. So we're doing better than what the patients have heard. But a lot of patients fear it's going to be 100%.

We are not promising them anything better than 50%, because if they're potent, great! Nobody is going to complain. But you hate to give false hope to people, especially someone who's older. They may be barely potent when they arrive, because of atherosclerosis; the blood supply to the pelvic area and the genitals may not be good because of blocked arteries. Their risk of becoming totally impotent is much higher.

Postscript

We just heard from a reliable source that, apparently due to intensive lobbying by special interest groups, Medicare does not, at this time, accept claims in connection with cryosurgery. It is expected, though, that by the time you read this, special "centers of excellence," such as the University of California Hospital in San Diego, Columbia-Presbyterian Hospital in New York, Allegheny General Hospital in Pittsburgh, and maybe others, will be accepted for reimbursement by Medicare.

There are, however, many cases where the cancer has already invaded too much surrounding tissue, or metastasized to other parts of the body, making it impossible to have a complete cure from cryosurgery alone. Dr. Nagourney tells us that in cases like this, where some time after cryosurgery the PSA (prostate specific antigen), a prostate cancer marker, starts going up again, he has had excellent results with putting these patients on intensive, short-term chemotherapy of only a week or so, followed by equally short-term radiation therapy.

Chapter 55

Benign Prostate Enlargement: Alternative Medical and Nutritional Therapies

There are nowadays only rare occasions where in the absence of cancer, surgery is indicated for merely benign prostate enlargement (BPE)—the frequent bane of men over fifty. In the more severe cases, the most frequently used surgical technique is still the traditional "transurethral" type of operation, in which parts of the enlarged prostate are cut away by inserting a cutting and viewing instrument through the urethra. In the hands of a highly skilled urologist, this delicate technique usually produces the desired results. More often than one would like to think and is generally admitted, though, this type of operation is not totally satisfactory and can result in serious side effects. (Your choice of the right surgeon is, hence, crucial.)

In most cases, though, medicine's first choice for BPE are newly developed, prostate-shrinking drugs like Proscar and Hytrin. Aside from that, there also are now very effective herbal remedies like saw palmetto and *Pygeum africanum* available, which even mainstream medicine is gradually coming around to acknowledging as safe and effective. (We accidentally discovered in the case of a friend, who was taking a prescription drug for BPE, that additional saw palmetto/*Pygeum africanum* as adjuct therapy, produced faster and better results than the prescription drug alone.)

In cases where prostate-shrinking drugs are, for one medical reason or another, less promising, there now also exists a device called the Prostatron that heats enlarged prostates with microwaves and thereby painlessly kills excess prostate tissue.

Just as cryosurgery represents a medical alternative to radical prostatectomy, the Prostatron technique represents an alternative medical therapy to transurethral surgery that is much less invasive and can be done with only local anesthesia. As the company making the Prostatron says, "a patient can have the procedure done in the morning, and be able to have dinner and watch the evening news at home."

Also, the Prostatron technique is much less expensive than the old-style transurethral operation, which costs between $8,000 and $12,000 and usually requires up to three days in the hospital. In contrast, the Prostatron technique costs less than half of that and usually does not cause such complications as impotence or incontinence. Its only downside is that in about a third of the men it may cause swelling that leaves them temporarily unable to urinate without a catheter.*

*Hospitals that use the Prostatron include Georgetown, Rush Presbyterian Hospital in Chicago, the Kidney Stone Center in Denver, and the Mayo Clinics in Rochester, Minnesota, and Jacksonville, Florida.

Part Ten

Macrobiotics

Chapter 56

The Macrobiotic Option

Of all nutritional regimens recommended for disease prevention in general, and cancer protection in particular, a macrobiotic diet seems especially worth considering. We therefore decided to look into macrobiotics in more detail, and here is what we found out.

A macrobiotic diet has its roots in traditional Japanese cooking and was introduced to America and Europe half a century ago by two of its principal teachers, George Ohsawa and Michio Kushi. But neither one actually invented the term "macrobiotic." Rather, it was coined over 150 years ago by the great German scientist and physician Wilhelm Hufeland, who used it for the title of his book *Makrobiotik—The Art of Prolonging Human Life*. Ohsawa simply borrowed the term and applied it to his own dietary system.

Ohsawa divided his basic diet into ten stages, from −3 to

+7, a system he called "Zen Macrobiotics" (in 1965 Ohsawa published a book of the same title). On each successive level, either the number of food items or the amounts allowed on the diet were reduced. On level 7, which Ohsawa considered most nearly ideal, the diet consisted almost totally of brown rice and other cereal grains.

Some people still follow Ohsawa's progressively more restrictive "Zen macrobiotics." Most practitioners of macrobiotics, however, use the more flexible and more inclusive type of diet developed by Michio Kushi, a former student of Ohsawa's who later came to overshadow him.

In Kushi's system, brown rice is still the basic item, supplemented by grains like barley, millet, oats, corn, rye, wheat, buckwheat (kasha), and more exotic grains like quinoa and amaranth. This single food category encompasses 50 to 60% of Kushi's macrobiotic diet. The rest includes:

25 to 30% vegetables (a third to be eaten raw, as in salads)
5 to 10% "seaweeds"
5 to 10% legumes (beans, especially Japanese azuki beans, lentils, garbanzos, etc.)

This basic diet is supplemented with soy products, such as tofu (unfermented soybean paste) and tempeh (fermented soybean paste).* At least 5% of all these basic foods (except fruits) are consumed as soups, mostly in the form of miso† soup, with the other foods added to it.

Occasional fish and scallops are allowed, but no shrimp and lobster or poultry or eggs.‡ Fruits are all right, provided they are locally grown in season. (Macrobiotics emphasizes that all fruits

*The best books on tofu (bean curd) and tempeh are by William Shurtleff and Akiko Aoyagi, published in 1979/1980, by Harper & Row.

†Miso, like tempeh, consists of the fermented and aged paste of soybeans, but the process of preparation is completely different (see Chapter 38).

‡Our own diet includes only egg whites, but no yolks because of their high cholesterol content (250 mg per yolk).

and vegetables must be consumed only in season and, if at all possible, grown locally.)

Since the macrobiotic diet is very low in sodium (only small amounts of sea salt are used), foods are often flavored with spices, as well as tamari and soy sauce. True, these sauces also have a relatively high sodium content, but since they are strongly flavored, smaller amounts are needed. Miso paste, which likewise has a high sea salt content, is also sometimes used for flavoring.

But the macrobiotic diet distinguishes itself as much by what is *not* supposed to be eaten as by what *can* be eaten. Forbidden foods on a macrobiotic "no-no" list include:

milk and other dairy products;
all chemically treated, highly salted, and processed foods;
red meat, poulty, eggs;
canned and frozen foods;
commercial fruit juices;
coffee and black tea;
refined sugar;
Coca-Cola, Pepsi-Cola, and all similar drinks;
iced drinks of any kind (only *green* tea and other herbal teas are allowed)

This is but a brief overview. A macrobiotic diet is far more complex and includes certain special combinations of foods and certain quasi-medicinal foods like pickled and aged umeboshi plums, shiitake mushrooms, and burdock root. There are several excellent books on the subject, so we need go no further into it here.

But macrobiotics is more than just diet and nutrition. It also represents a certain holistic world view, centered in nonviolence and ecological concerns, harmony with nature, "reverence for life," meditation, and so on; in short, macrobiotics represents a spiritual, nonmaterialistic orientation to life, which we are much in favor of.

It follows that macrobiotic philosophy considers disease,

and especially cancer, to be the result of eating the wrong food, being out of harmony with nature, of having the wrong lifestyle and the wrong mental attitudes. In fact, we think these philosophical and psychological factors—along with group support—can take as much credit as diet for the often remarkably beneficial results obtained by macrobiotics.

Macrobiotic thinking, however, places less emphasis on these things and attributes the current increase in cancer and other chronic diseases as being primarily due to wrong diet, with other factors playing only secondary roles. For that reason, Kushi is convinced—in our view, rightly—that "a macrobiotically balanced diet may positively influence the outcome of existing cancers."*

As it happens, we know of a case that seems to corroborate Michio Kushi's statement, a case we will present in the following chapter. But first this brief introduction:

In 1990, Alan M. Kapuler was diagnosed with mixed cell lymphoma. It so happened that he was a friend of the same friends of ours in San Diego, the Drs. Sheldon and Joyce Hendler, who referred him to Dr. Robert Nagourney for medical advice, just as they had referred Eberhard to him, when he was first (falsely) diagnosed with multiple myeloma.

So it was that Dr. Kapuler consulted with Dr. Nagourney about a possible chemotherapy for his cancer. Dr. Nagourney, as the reader will recall (see Chapters 51, 52, and 53), believes in "customizing" chemotherapy, rather than treating all patients who have the same kind of cancer with the same chemotherapy drugs. For that reason, he insists that, whenever possible, a certain laboratory test be conducted.

In Dr. Kapuler's case, unfortunately, the patient's cancer cells proved resistant to everything but a particularly vicious chemical compound, nitrogen mustard, a relative of mustard gas, a nerve poison of World War I notoriety. Obviously that kind of therapy did not appeal to Dr. Kapuler, who knew of the likelihood of very unpleasant side effects. What made him even

*As cited in Ralph Moss, *Cancer Therapy,* 196.

more reluctant to use this highly toxic chemotherapy was that medical statistics have shown that even this was not likely to buy him more than seven years. So he said, "No, thanks!" and started looking elsewhere.

After considering several "alternative" cancer therapies, he opted for macrobiotics, plus the so-called "Hoxsey tonic," made of nine medicinal plant extracts, plus potassium iodide. Moreover, he has chronicled his experiences with this combination of macrobiotics and herbal therapy over the past three years and published them in his own biological research journal, *Peace Seeds Research Journal.*

Firsthand accounts like this, especially from a scientifically trained observer, are rare. We are therefore grateful to Dr. Kapuler for letting us present his story in the chapters that follow.

We also recommend the following books if you are considering macrobiotics, in general, or as adjunct cancer treatment.

RECOMMENDED READING

Esko, Edward, ed. *Doctors Look at Macrobiotics*. NY: Japan Publishing Co., 1988.

Faulkne, Hugh. *Physician Heal Thyself.* Becket, MA: One Peaceful World Press, 1992.

Kushi, Aveline. *Macrobiotic Cooking*. Warner Books, NY: 1985.

Kushi, Michio. *The Cancer Prevention Diet*. St. Martin's Press, NY: 1983.

Nussbaum, E. *Recovery from Cancer to Health Through Macrobiotics*. NY: Japan Publishing Co., 1986 (reprint by Avery Publishing Grp., Garden City, NY).

Ohsawa, George. *Macrobiotics: The Way of Healing*. Ohsawa Fdn., Oroville, CA, 1981.

Chapter 57

Recovery from Lymphatic Cancer: A Tribute to Macrobiotics by Alan M. Kapuler, Ph.D.*

The sunlight coming through the greenhouse roof was warming my heart and reminding me once again of how beautiful life is on earth.

Only a year ealier I had been wondering about years to live, looking at my wife and daughters' faces, as if each time for the last time. The reality of swollen lumps in my groin, in my neck, and under my arms had come home to me: lymphatic cancer.

Impossible. I could not believe it. At twenty-six when I weighed 192 pounds, I stopped eating meat, and at thirty-one,

*This text represents an edited and slightly abridged version of Dr. Alan M. Kapuler's orginal article in *Peace Seeds Research Journal,* vol. 6, 1991, by permission of Dr. Alan M. Kapuler. Those interested in obtaining the *Peace Seeds* journal should write to: Peace Seeds, 2385 SE Thompson St., Corvallis, OR 97333-1919.

chicken and fish. By age forty-seven, I was 145 pounds, having been a lacto-ovo vegetarian for sixteen years and eating organic foods for about as long.

It was in August, after long days of weeding and harvesting seed crops [Dr. Kapuler now operates an organic seed company], that I noticed that some of my lymph nodes were quite large . . . abnormally large. For a while I put ice packs on them to see if it would stop their growth. The ice packs were alternated with a heating pad. The process had no effect, so I began drinking lots of ginger tea. It didn't seem to help either.

A few weeks later I flew to La Jolla, California, to visit Dr. Sheldon Hendler, a longtime friend. For several decades we have shared the language of the molecules and used it to improve the human condition, to make sense of sickness by understanding how the molecules and the cells they build actually work.

He had arranged for a standard set of tests, including a whole body scan, blood and urine analysis, a complete physical exam, and finally a biopsy. For a while we hoped for an obscure fungal disorder that causes swollen lymph glands. Then we hoped for a simple kind of leukemia with a high survival rate. Leukemia, after all, was a distinct possibility; I had often been wondering if my years as a molecular biologist and, in particular, the time I spent working with avian leukemia and sarcoma viruses would come back to haunt me. Now I was almost hoping that it would do so.

But when my lymph node tissue, analyzed under a microscope, showed several cell types characteristic of a mixed cell lymphoma, the prognosis wasn't so good. My heart would speed up and echo in my chest, and I would get the dull, mind-reducing ache of worry about my wife, my life, my kids, and who was going to pay the bills.

For eight and a half months, the lymph nodes remained swollen but didn't increase in number or in size, and it was during this period that I recollected how bad I had felt after the biopsy. It had involved only the surgical removal of two of the swollen lymph nodes. But the surgeon insisted on taking also some of the surrounding tissue to make sure there was enough to work with for further tests.

It would have made sense—if I hadn't known that there were many millions of cells in a lymph node. Anyway, after the operation I was sore, hunched over, severely depressed, and in a partially destroyed state that marked the physical low point of my cancer experience.

It takes two weeks to recover from the pain of as simple an operation as the removal of two inguinal lymph nodes. I didn't know that two years ago, but I know it now. For months I stared at the swollen nodes that looked like quail eggs, snagging my hands when I'd rub my neck or chest. It gave me rushes of intense self-hatred. I worked on my anger about the injustice of cancer. I was ignorant, didn't know how to feed myself, didn't know how to choose from Safeway's grand aisles the occasional product in thousands that would be all right to eat.

In the wake of the biopsy was the chemscan data on my own cells. After taking out the lymph nodes to analyze for malignant cells, some of the cells were cultured and their sensitivity toward several kinds of cancer cell poisons tested. They found that mustard gas would be the most effective chemotherapeutic poison. I asked Dr. Hendler about my life expectancy (if I took the chemotherapy), and he said, seven years. So I figured there was some time to look for other ways to heal.

Here I was, I had lymphatic cancer, and needed a cure. I knew that part of getting well had to do with how I felt about myself. Another part of getting well had to do with what and how I eat. They interconnect in important and specific ways. So I began searching for a way to promote my own healing.

> "The proper place to perform cancer surgery is not in the operating room after the disease has run its course, but in the kitchen and in other areas of daily life before it has developed."
>
> —Michio Kushi, *The Cancer Prevention Diet*

The first thing that went through my mind was to give up all sources of stress, particularly in the diet. So my lacto-ovo-vegetarian diet was due for an overhaul. So was my timing and pattern of eating.

I had many suggestions for healing regimens to follow. For instance, a friend sent me a mattress made of small magnets with a cover and pillow, both of which also contained magnets. It is said to help with cancer and many other diseases. I have been sleeping on it for most of the last thirteen months and find it very comfortable. But it could only be a small aid in the much larger, more fundamental, nontoxic therapy I was looking for.

Perhaps for the same reasons that led me to leave Eastern academia in the early 1970s, head out West to find family and friends, organic gardening, and the gene pool of edible plants, I decided to find out some more about cancer cures and nontoxic approaches to healing.

After getting back from La Jolla as a cancer patient, my wonderful and devoted wife, Linda, made changes in the kitchen. Ohsawa relates that "the fundamental material for the factory of married life that produces happiness is food."*

We had read several accounts of recovery from terminal and metastatic cancer by virtue of a dietary regime called macrobiotics.† Following Michio Kushi's analysis of lymphatic cancer in *The Cancer Prevention Diet*, and Aveline Kushi's recipes in *Macrobiotic Cooking*, we began to change.

I had vowed to give up rather cherished but unhealthy habits like tobacco (I rolled my own for sixteen years), and my very sweet and white coffee in the morning. But I hadn't reckoned what it would be like without bread, honey, cheese, fruits, fresh salads, tomatoes, potatoes, eggplants, peppers, oils, and pizza.

I had yet to see the intimacy of the sugar connection in

*Ohsawa, G. *Macrobiotic Guidebook for Living*. Ohsawa Fdn., Oroville, CA; 1985.

†Ohsawa, G. *Macrobiotics: The Way of Healing*. Ohsawa Fdn., Oroville, CA; 1981.

the control of so many of our lives; Dufty's book *Sugar Blues* helped me with that.* Shurtleff and Aoyagi's great books on tofu, tempeh, and miso† renewed my connections between biochemistry and food, between nutrition and molecules, and stimulated the search for free amino acids in our vegetables as a common feature of nutrition.

For the first few months, having changed some major aspects of my intake of food, I felt good. The nodes were there, but they weren't getting larger and there were no new ones. In one of Kushi's books, it is said that if you befriend your cancer it will become your best friend. My nodes had rocked me out of a destructive life pattern and mindset, had turned me from vanity to humility, from isolated egotism to a sense of universal connectedness, love, and compassion. I was grateful to understand, grateful for a supportive family, and glad to shed some longtime cherished behaviors like the midnight snack. (In macrobiotics one waits three to four hours after eating before sleeping.) Also, after many years of erratic and minimal breakfasts, I now eat rice or whole oats in the morning.

There are so many things to learn when starting out on the macrobiotic path. I reasoned that since I had lymphatic cancer, I had to drop any pretense of knowledge. I was glad for guidance. Jensei and Kazuko Yamasake, two macrobiotic counselors, provided it at difficult times by providing organic miso and umeboshi [preserved Japanese plum], both essential nutritional components of the dietary system. More important yet, they taught me the wisdom of patience.

I began with the notion of adhering to the regimen for at least a year, but by the seventh month, the nodes were still swollen, the same size as when I started, and I began to consider the use of herbs. I liked the notion of using herbs to get well from cancer. I grew several of the best known kinds and had seeds for others. But, at the time, I decided that to mix therapies would make it difficult later on. So I continued, for the time

*Dufty, W., *Sugar Blues*. NY: Warner Books, 1975.
†Shurtleff, W. and A. Aoyagi, *The Book of Miso*. Japan: Autumn Press, 1976.

being, with just the macrobiotic regimen, but paid more attention to chewing thoroughly and was grateful for organic, short-grain brown rice.

By midsummer, the seed harvesting season on our farm was well under way, the workload prodigious, and after figuring that I needed a light year to concentrate on getting the nodes to return to normal, I found myself with even more work than usual. Among other things, I had to give a lecture at a conference in Santa Fe. It took months to prepare the talk. My friend and co-worker Gurusiddhia and I had new data on free amino acids, adding snap beans, okra, and sweet corn as excellent sources.

Of course, the airlines don't offer macrobiotic food, but I brought my own rice rolls in sushi nori (sticky rice, wrapped in thin sheets of dried seaweed) on the flight to Santa Fe. In Santa Fe, my search for macrobiotic foods led me to the discovery of a fine restaurant specializing in macrobiotic-like cuisine. I especially remember a delicious red sauce, called nomato, that looked like tomato, but actually was a mix of beet and carrot. So I learned, once again, that all macrobiotics demands of us is to attend to our own healing. If we do that, we will always find opportunities to eat the macrobiotic way, no matter where we are.

After returning from the conference, refreshed from having had an enthusiastic reception, I realized that I wasn't noticing my lymph nodes as much as before. I suspected that they were smaller, but didn't want to comment on it, not even to myself. But by my birthday, in early September, I got the best present ever: the nodes were clearly going down, and by mid-October they were normal.

An oncologist had been following my progress from soon after the biopsy until the nodes returned to normal. He had occasionally urged me to take chemotherapy. I had the impression that he had never seen a remission of a mixed cell lymphoma. It just didn't happen. Yet, I had related to him from the outset that I was practicing a rather strict macrobiotic regimen which had an impressive success rate for sending cancers into remission. During the sequence of visits where he examined and measured the nodes and took blood for cell and enzyme analyses, he told me that remission caused by radiation and chemotherapy generally lasts for several years and then the nodes swell up again.

The current medical practices of poisoning the cancers, if not ourselves, or cutting them out surgically, do not deal with the origins of cancer. We treat symptoms and not causes. By associating them with viruses and genetic events in the chromosomes of our cells, we never reach the essential nutritional causality. As a society, too, we have lost contact with the greater cycle of feeding and nutrition of the web of living organisms. This is demonstrated by our monocultural and poison-based agriculture, which we are so proud of. So on several levels we deny the contribution of nutrition to our health and happiness.

Anyway, my lymph nodes were normal and I felt blessed by the courageous souls who had insisted that the body will heal itself, given the right food. And an important part of the right food is *less* food and an understanding of balance, of duality in unity, of yin and yang, of acid and alkaline, of DNA and the genetic code.

From the outset, my molecular scientific training told me that chemotherapy and radiation were poisonous and destructive. The notion that we can kill disease, just as we kill cattle, has disgraced our society for generations. We've become licensed experts on poison. We need more experts on regrowing broken ecosystems. We need more experts on diversity.

During my first complete year practicing macrobiotics, I didn't get a virus, flu, or cold, as I had several times a year for many years. I could feel the beginnings but somehow they never took. By the next day, I was fine. Only after these experiences have I recognized that by not feeding sweets, oils, high-protein foods, fruit juices, and bread to my body, these foodstuffs of ill health are not available for the viruses and bacteria to feed on. Measured by heart, kidney, liver, pancreatic and lung disease, as well as cancer, our bodies clearly don't heal well eating what we normally eat. Macrobiotics simplifies, streamlines, and changes the diet. In the process, there is time to heal.

In my childhood, nobody ate anything like a rice-centered diet. There were no models of a holistic kitchen. Whole grains weren't even a rumor. Salad was for women. My father reigned as chief carnivore, surrounded by the grandpas. Medicine meant penicillin. And with the antibiotics came orange juice, just as after the tonsils are removed you get ice cream. Amazing how long it takes to understand that the sugar feeds the bacteria growing in the tonsils. And why are the viruses growing in the swollen lymph nodes? Because of our food system. Because of what I had eaten and because of what my mother had eaten when I was in her womb.

I had reflected frequently about the role of sugars from plant foods, but hadn't insisted that if one is going to drop sugar, it means fruit sugar and cane sugar and date sugar and beet sugar and corn sugar and insect sugar—*any* kind of sugar! How we bribe our kids with sweet treats and then discover behavior problems.

On the other hand, the starch in the rice seed is made of a kind of sugar too, but of a totally different kind. Complex carbohydrates like rice are polymers, or forerunners, of sweet sugar. So are cellulose and glycogen, with all of which our bodies can cope much better than with the sweet sugars themselves. One central issue in transforming the nutritional value of our food system therefore is to create a better balance between the small, sweet sugar molecules, like glucose and fructose, to which we are so addicted, and their healthier complex polymers, like the starch in grains.

A comparable area of investigation is the balance of free amino acids and their polymers, the proteins, which are so dominant in our diet. Our American society has increasingly favored a high-protein, meat-centered diet, producing overeating carnivores. It has created giants, but are we slim, good-humored, and healthy as a society?

It is several months since the lymph nodes have returned

to normal. My health and vigor are excellent. Participating in a yoga class has helped. Our household continues its course in macrobiotics. My only physical symptom is that I have a chronic rash on one finger that I can't get rid of. Perhaps it is to remind me that I must continue on the journey of healing my body.

When I was thirty, I threw away my eyeglasses. Now, as my eyesight goes through changes, I have begun macrobiotic practices for maintaining clear and accurate vision. As in each dramatic step towards self-realization we know that we have turned another corner, so the transformations of our physical being are immediately before us all.

Lymphoma demanded that I pay attention to being fully alive. Macrobiotics continues this focus and its unfolding.

Addendum

It is now almost five months since the lymph nodes have returned to normal size. My health has been improving steadily and I continue to practice and enjoy the macrobiotic dietary regimen, although I am not as exacting as during the months when my focus was recovering from lymphatics cancer.

My focus has changed from the lymphatics to my liver and kidneys. As discussed in *How to See Your Health: Book of Oriental Diagnosis* by Michio Kushi (Japan Publications, 1980), "reading" the face and body develops insight about the health of our internal organs. The strong creases between my eyebrows are associated with a stressed liver and are known as liver pain and anger lines. The liver has a major role in the turnover of blood cells, so the return of lymphatics to normal has required extra work by the liver.

I still find that living in a society that values profit before people, pesticide-maintained fields to rare species, and coercion instead of cooperation, raises my bile—a phrase relating to the gall bladder, which is surrounded by the liver. Rather than reinforcing anger toward the common injustices that surround me, I am working toward ways of sharing concern about our diets, our agricultural practices, and the way we are educated.

During the year when I visited a local oncologist, my blood chemistry was analyzed bimonthly. The results were normal for all categories, and the most striking observation was that subsequent to adhering to the macrobiotic diet, my cholesterol level dropped to a very low yet normal reading. This reinforced the understanding that the macrobiotic food system works to promote healing not only from cancer but from heart disease as well.

I have been fortunate to have the support of a loving wife and family during the recent difficult years. They have followed a comparable though less strict dietary regime. We have been virtually free from the common colds and bronchitis that troubled us previously. Collectively our health has been wonderful and we gratefully thank everyone who has contributed to the science of macrobiotics.

Chapter 58

A Healing During Corn Season by Alan M. Kapuler, Ph.D.*

After three and a half years of remission from lymphatic cancer, thanks to being eleven months on a 5+ Ohsawa macrobiotic diet, my neck suddenly thickened up again in January 1993. Looking back, I think I know why it happened. For one thing, I was worried about money and had been under a lot of other work-related stress.† Furthermore, I had eaten sev-

*By permission of the author, Dr. Alan M. Kapuler. The original text of this article appear in *Peace Seeds*, vol. 7, 1994. This is an edited and slightly abridged version. Those interested in obtaining a copy of *Peace Seeds Research Journal* should write to Peace Seeds, 2385 SE Thompson St., Corvallis, OR 97333–1919.

†Dr. Alan Kapuler runs a highly sophisticated, organic seed business called Peace Seeds, in Corvallis, Oregon. He specializes in vegetable seeds with the highest content of free amino acids and hence optimum nutritional value. Peace Seeds are carried by some health food stores, or can be ordered directly from Dr. Kapuler's company, Peace Seeds.

eral ounces of a very sweet holiday confection—something that certainly was *not* on my macrobiotic diet.

Two days later I had a gum infection, accompanied by a one-inch swollen lymph gland that was sore and painful to touch. I took standard penicillin-type antibiotics, and it slowly receded in ten days. Two weeks later, I had a sore left ear with a double deposit of earwax, one part around the auditory canal and the other directly on the tympanic membrane, making it very sensitive to touch.

I used olive oil and other oil softeners, but finally found that warm glycerol and hydrogen peroxide worked best. I used a small, low-pressure hand syringe to rinse out the ear once or twice daily for a week. After a couple of days' break, I did it again and a dime-sized wax plug came out of my ear. After that, my ear no longer hurt, but the infection that came from the earwax plugging the ear canal had caused six lymph nodes to become enlarged. The trouble was that when the ear cleared up, the nodes did not go back to normal size. I had lymphoma again.

This time it was much easier to admit to myself that I had lymphatic cancer than it was when I initially encountered my swollen glands four years previously. Nor was it hard to find out why it had happened. I had not been as strict with my diet during remission as I had been when I was actively seeking a natural cancer cure. It was a fall from grace after a wonderful success at self-healing.

Nonetheless, I had basically stayed on a macrobiotic diet, because I enjoy the simplicity and depth of a diet based on rice, vegetables, and miso soup. Several times friends and associates would be provoked by the apparent boredom and repetitiousness of my daily food intake, but to me, each apparently identical bowl of rice is unique.

I am perfectly happy to eat miso soup, rice, and a few veggies for breakfast and lunch. Dinner includes more vegetables and usually cooked beans, especially azuki beans, but also garbanzos, lentils, tempeh, or tofu. Other parts of the daily diet are sushi nori (sticky rice wrapped in a paper-thin piece of dried seaweed), hijiki or other seaweed, and an umeboshi plum or two. I am particularly careful to eat organically grown grains and produce. But, as said earlier, I had become a little lax during the remission and now I was being handed the bill.

Finding myself with lymphoma again, I consulted several physicians with diverse approaches. Two of them were regular M.D.s, one was an M.D. and Ph.D., another one an N.D. (doctor of naturopathy), and there was also a Chinese acupuncturist and a macrobiotic counselor. In addition, I went to the Bio-Medical Center in Tijuana, Mexico, where they prescribe the Hoxsey herbal tonic.* After meeting these healers, my diet and outlook changed. Most delightful was the return of raw garlic, a clove or two at every meal. I also added some flaxseed oil (high in gamma linoleic acid) and, for a while, 200 units of vitamin E per day. At the same time, I expanded my grain base to include more millet, quinoa, amaranth, and long-grain brown rice, while decreasing my heavy reliance on short-grain brown rice.

It was also suggested that my diet be less rigid and include some almonds, pumpkin and sunflower seeds, and occasional baked apples as snacks, as well as more steamed greens, particularly mustards, kale, and dandelion, but I was advised to avoid tomatoes and vinegar.† I continue to have acupuncture treatments and am drinking a sequence of Chinese medicinal teas, to which I added one to three cups of Pau D'arco tea daily.‡

*The "Hoxsey tonic" consists of nine herbal extracts plus potassium iodide salts from Nettle Leaf. A similar though not identical version of this herbal mixture can be obtained from Gaia Herbs (1-800-831-7780), but is called "Hoxsey Red Clover Supreme."

†The warning about tomatoes and vinegar probably came from nurse Mildred Nelson, director of the Bio-Medical Center in Tijuana, Mexico (Hoxsey clinic). Her well-known prohibition of tomatoes for her patients is all the more questionable in light of the recent discoveries concerning the protective effect of lycopene from tomatoes, especially with regard to prostate cancer.

‡Lapachol, the principal active ingredient in Pau D'arco, appears indeed to have anticancer properties. The problem, however, is that what little research exists on Pau D'arco makes it doubtful whether small amounts of it (as in one to three cups of tea) are really effective, whereas higher doses may be too toxic.

The first time my lymphoma receded, I had been feasting on fresh sweet corn, a crop rich in free amino acids and good for lymphatic circulation. The second remission began with the start of corn season and progressed well enough to be normal by September.

It was during that period that I went to Tijuana to talk to "Nurse Mildred" and the doctors at the Bio-Medical Center (Hoxsey clinic). My doctor there said I was, apart from the lymphoma recurrence, basically in excellent health, which he attributed to my diet. He had no doubt that, if I continued with my diet and took the Hoxsey tonic, the lymph nodes would return to normal within two months.

As I write this, it is fourteen months since I first visited the clinic. The lymph nodes have been normal for twelve months, so the doctor at the Center was right on the button. Remission has taken four months this time, rather than eleven months the first time, when I followed strict macrobiotic guidelines, but without the Hoxsey tonics.

After the swollen lymph nodes receded the first time, an irritating rash developed on my right hand. At the place where the digits meet the palm, little glassy bubbles would arise in waves and spread between the fingers. They would harden and crack and sometimes ooze fluid. As the bubbles increased in number, the skin became so sore and raw that, after a few months, I found it too painful to close my hand. Bach's topical herbal rescue remedy was the best palliative, offering some relief. But it was only after six months that the waves of bubbles receded and the hand became usable again. It took a couple of years more for the skin to soften up and regain its normal resiliency and texture.

After the lymph nodes had returned to normal, the rash appeared on my hand once again. This time it was milder, appearing and disappearing in about six weeks. What helped was the fresh juice from aloe vera leaves. The aloe promoted healing in a rapid and dramatic way, better than any other remedy. Kazuko Yamasake, my macrobiotics advisor, said that the healing moves from inside out—from the spleen and internal lymphatics to the skin—in my case, the hand being one of the last organs to become whole and healthy again.

When the lymph nodes swelled up the second time, I was asked if I wanted another biopsy. I replied that it did not matter whether the swollen glands were lymphatic cancer, or whether they were caused by a virus. My system obviously was out of balance and I was out of touch with my center. I definitely was in need of some more work on myself.

I am increasingly aware of stress. I see it as an assault on my pituitary, shocks to my immune system, attacks on my internal sense of well-being. On the other hand, I realize that—regardless of our outward circumstances—we can make ourselves sick and can heal ourselves as well. But although I strive to accurately and thoroughly elicit a centered response to all circumstances, I find my ability to heal myself is rather limited and in strong need of cultivation.

The one thing that I find most useful and perhaps essential in that respect is macrobiotics, both as diet and philosophy. Naturally, the diet is responsive to our personal condition, the sum of physical, mental, and spiritual energies that we manifest. But I know, it is ultimately up to me to be letting go of my body, my ego, and the misinformed voices of fear and insecurity that still sometimes intrude into my consciousness.

I have no doubt that some of our physical and social problems come from the long history of violence and murderous misdeeds that have entered, DNA-like, into our system. Some progress towards *ahimsa* (nonviolence) is therefore urgently needed for the longterm sustainability of our species.

Several years ago, when I noticed swollen lymph glands in my neck, chest, and groin, it had not occurred to me that the journey of moments that make a day, and the days that mark the earth's yearly passage around the sun, would find macrobiotics at the center of my daily prayer for peace and love. Today, I am convinced that if macrobiotics succeeds in producing a continuous flow of healed people living in harmony and self-awareness, a new food system will emerge and our society will undergo a profound transformation.

This is my message and my prayer, both for the healing of myself and for the planet, which has become sick with our own sickness.

Index